What people

Coo

By far the most accessible and practical book on love and sex that I've ever read. As I was reading it, I felt myself changing positively, without even doing anything! Having already experienced the incredible power of mindfulness in so many other ways, I need no convincing that by applying the recommendations here, you'll witness your relationship with sex transform bringing greater pleasure, loving kindness and intimacy. It's motivated me to continue deepening my mindfulness practice into the sexual sphere. I wholeheartedly recommend this inspiring book to young adults. **Darren Cockburn**, author of internationally acclaimed *Being Present* and *Living a Life of Harmony*

Cool Sex is a generous and expert guide to loving and fulfilling sex for young adults. This book arises from decades of Diana's exploration into the profound relaxation, intimacy and deep pleasure states available through cool sex, and from guiding many thousands of couples and individuals to explore these transformative experiences for themselves. I'm thrilled that in *Cool Sex* Diana and Wendy are now offering this practical instruction and timeless wisdom to young adults from the beginning of their sexual journey, and in such a clear, warm, inclusive and respectful way. What a beautiful and accessible antidote to disconnection, dissatisfaction, stress and anxiety in relationships and in life. What a gift!
Jane Bennet, Puberty educator and author of several books including *The Pill: Are You Sure It's for You?*

Cool Sex

An essential young adult guide
to loving, fulfilling sex

Cool Sex

An essential young adult guide
to loving, fulfilling sex

Diana Richardson
& Wendy Doeleman

BOOKS

Winchester, UK
Washington, USA

JOHN HUNT PUBLISHING

First published by O-Books, 2020
O-Books is an imprint of John Hunt Publishing Ltd., 3 East St., Alresford,
Hampshire SO24 9EE, UK
office@jhpbooks.com
www.johnhuntpublishing.com
www.o-books.com

For distributor details and how to order please visit the 'Ordering' section on our website.

Text copyright: Diana Richardson & Wendy Doeleman 2019

ISBN: 978 1 78904 351 8
978 1 78904 352 5 (ebook)
Library of Congress Control Number: 2019948227

A CIP catalogue record for this book is available from the British Library.

Design: Stuart Davies

UK: Printed and bound by CPI Group (UK) Ltd, Croydon, CR0 4YY
Printed in North America by CPI GPS partners

We operate a distinctive and ethical publishing philosophy in all areas of our business, from our global network of authors to production and worldwide distribution.

Contents

Titles by Diana Richardson

The Heart of Tantric Sex.
A Unique Guide to Love and Sexual Fulfilment
Diana Richardson, O-Books, UK. 2003
ISBN 978-1-90381-637-8

Tantric Orgasm for Women
Diana Richardson, Destiny Books, USA. 2004
ISBN 978-0-89281-133-5

Tantric Love: Feeling vs Emotion. Golden rules to make love easy
Diana & Michael Richardson, O-Books, UK. 2004
ISBN 978-1-84694-283-9

Tantric Sex for Men: Making Love a Meditation
Diana & Michael Richardson, Destiny Books, USA. 2010
ISBN 978-1-59477-311-2

Slow Sex. The Path to Fulfilling and Sustainable Sexuality
Diana Richardson, Destiny Books, USA. 2011
ISBN 978-1-59477-367-9

Tantric Love Letters: On Sex and Affairs of the Heart
Diana Richardson, O-Books, UK. 2011
ISBN 978-1-78099-154-2

Tantric Sex and Menopause. Practices for Spiritual and Sexual Renewal
Diana Richardson & Janet McGeever, Destiny Books, USA. 2018
ISBN 978-1-62055-683-2

To the well-being of our future generations

Preface by Diana Richardson

Cool Sex is written specifically with young adults in mind, age range 15–25 years. Even so, one mother reported to me that her son of 14 read the German edition, and he basically "swallowed the contents" and seemed very happy! So, ultimately it will depend on the individual.

It's for sure an informative read for older adults too. In the week-long Making Love Retreats for couples that I lead together with my partner Michael, the German and French editions of this book are on display and I notice many participants reading it in a highly engaged way – age range 25–75!

From my perspective age is of no consequence when it comes to the sexual material in this book (or any of my previous books), because as a society we are not truly informed about sex. We believe that sex should be instinctive and that we should know 'how' to do it. However, we have more or less lost contact with our original true instinct and have been sexually 'imprinted' to behave in certain ways in sex. And these ways are handed down, generation to generation.

So in the long run basically all of us are affected – to a greater or lesser degree – by a limited view of sex and its many misunderstandings. And in this sense age does not matter – because as far as sex goes – we are all much on the same page.

Cool Sex provides alternative information that is grounded in the physical and energetic realities of the body. It is a shift away from building up intensity and excitement – the heat of sex – to the cooler zones of sex using relaxation and awareness (mindfulness). Discovering and exploring the other side of the sexual coin delivers deeper sexual satisfaction and fulfilment and also creates love and harmony.

Over the last twenty-five years of working with couples, frequently at the end of the retreats, parents ask, "How can we inform our children about a different style of sex? We don't want them to wait – like we had to – until they are 40/50 years old to find out about it." Parents realize that it would probably have saved them a lot of problems to have known about a viable sexual alternative when they were *a lot* younger – a style that encourages love and connection. *Cool Sex* represents a summary of the information shared with adults during this week-long retreat.

I am very grateful to Wendy Doeleman for our creative collaboration over the years, and especially for her unique way of attuning the information to a younger audience. We met in a Making Love Retreat in 2009 which inspired Wendy to write the original version of *Cool Sex – Coole seks, relaxte liefde* – published in Dutch in 2010. We are thrilled that now this book – in its revised and expanded form – is available in English.

Diana Richardson

Acknowledgements

We extend our appreciation and gratitude to Gina Qualliotine and Ammy Mamolito from the USA, for their encouragement and generous support in giving birth to this our English edition of *Cool Sex*.

Our warm-hearted thanks to Roman Korver from the Netherlands, who at the age of 19 (in 2009) drew the diagrams that appear in this book (Figures 2–6). We are delighted to have this opportunity to share them with others.

We are deeply indebted and grateful to our publishers O-Books – an imprint of John Hunt Publishers – for their far-reaching vision and commitment to the well-being of our future generations.

Disclaimer

The guidance and suggestions given in this book are to be the personal choice and wish of any individual, young or old, and should there be any issues relating to health, please consult a doctor or a therapist. Neither we the authors nor the publisher accept any responsibility for any consequences of a reader failing to take appropriate health advice.

List of Illustrations with page numbers

Fig. 1 taken from page 20 – *The Heart of Tantric Sex* by Diana Richardson
Fig. 2, 3, 4, 5, 6 – Illustrations by Roman Korver, Netherlands. Copyright 2009.

List of Exercises with page numbers

Chapter 1

What Is True?

Test your knowledge about sex!
Which of the following statements are true in your opinion?

- ☐ In order to have sexual intercourse a guy has to have a hard-on (an erection).
- ☐ The clitoris is the main source of pleasure for a girl.
- ☐ For sex to be good the guy must have a hard-on for a long time.
- ☐ If sex becomes boring, it is good to increase stimulation and excitement.
- ☐ A tight vagina and a big penis give the most pleasure during sex.
- ☐ The point of foreplay is to get more and more excited.
- ☐ If a guy has an orgasm, it means he ejaculates.
- ☐ For sex to be good there must be a lot of movement.
- ☐ For sex to be good you both have to 'cum' (have an orgasm).
- ☐ To have sex you need to get excited and as 'hot' as possible.

What is the truth?
So, how many times did you answer true? Probably several times, since these are statements that many people think are true. Yet as you will learn in this book there is another way to have sex. It's called cool sex, and from the perspective of cool sex all of the statements are not necessarily true. Although some of the information in this book will sound new to many people, it is in fact drawn from ancient wisdom called neo-tantra.

Who is this book written for?

Cool Sex is suitable for all young adults. For those who have some sexual experience and are curious to discover more; and for those wanting to find out 'something different' about sex before they start out.

Waiting for marriage?

Cool Sex is also of value for couples who choose to wait for religious reasons or personal reasons, to have sex after marriage; it can be an orientation and preparation for their future sex life. Some of the suggested exercises can be done alone, and others can be done together while fully clothed.

Gender themes and sexual combinations

In this book we use the words guy/boy and girl quite often, and by this we mean the male-female combination. At the same time, there are some of us who are attracted to the same gender as ourselves, some of us who feel gender fluid and others who identify with a gender different to the one they were born with.

There are many words used to describe different sexual combinations. Words we hear, for example, are heterosexual, hetero, straight, homosexual, gay, lesbian, bisexual, queer and asexual. Even so, some individuals feel that the term used to describe their category does not necessarily connect with their inner feeling.

In the end cool sex is suitable for everyone because, as will be explained in Chapter 3, every person carries feminine and masculine energies. This means each individual can play with both of these energies and qualities in their own way.

We highly recommend that the information in this book is adapted to fit your personal situation. The general approach of cool sex can definitely be applied and explored by all lovers!

A journey of exploration

Reading a book is one thing, but the actual experience of cool sex is something else. If you really want to experience what this kind of sex involves, you can try out the ideas and exercises suggested in this book. Some of them you can do on your own. Others are done together with a partner. Experimenting with cool sex is like an open-ended adventure with no set destination. Let yourself be surprised by what you discover and experience along the way.

Chapter 2

Is Sex Hot?

We think sex is meant to be hot – the hotter the better. Just look around you – at video clips, on the Internet, along the street, watching movies, in commercials, at the bus stop and in magazines. Half-naked bodies, inviting postures and suggestive messages are to be seen everywhere! This is not, of course, for no reason. Sex for most people is exciting, interesting, attractive, even sometimes truly irresistible, and because of this sex has the power to sell things.

Hot variety is common

Most of the images we see show a type of sex that is hot. In other words, there is some level of enticement, stimulation, excitement and intensity. And eventually, this can include stimulation of your own genitals, or another's genitals, with or without physical penetration.

Almost everyone who has experienced sex probably knows the hot variety of sex. This style is usually pretty purposeful and focused in how it is done because there is the intention to reach orgasm – it's like the goal of sex, it's the reason to have sex.

By increasing stimulation and excitement to an intense level it is possible to bring the sensations to a climax – almost as a form of tension – that peaks and discharges pleasurably through the genitals in a few seconds of orgasm.

After this happens the excitement and interest will fall away very quickly and usually means that sex, for now, is over. Hot sex can take place in an atmosphere of love, but it can also take place without love where the heart is uninvolved in the experience.

Sex with intimacy

The expression making love (and lovemaking) seem to be words that are usually used to describe another kind of sexual exchange. For many people these words will mean hugging, kissing, caressing, massaging and intimately being together in a loving, peaceful atmosphere. But making love doesn't necessarily mean that there is penetration with lots of excitement.

Even so hot sex and lovemaking are, of course, not always so different. Especially when you are in love you naturally combine hot sex with kissing, fondling, caressing, talking, laughing, crying and so on. In short this means that through sex you can also experience real intimacy together. However, the tendency is to view this as soft love, more as a type of foreplay which often, if not always, is considered to be just a way to get to the real thing, namely hot sex.

The downsides of hot sex

For sure hot sex can be very pleasurable and can become a favorite interest for many people. And, if it is not happening in actual practice then it can be happening in thought or fantasy. However, experience shows us that there are also some downsides to hot sex.

Here are some of the things that can be related to hot sex:

◆ Premature ejaculation.
◆ No orgasm or difficulty in reaching an orgasm.
◆ Obsession with or addiction to sex and/or masturbation, with or without porn.
◆ Pain during sex or after sex.
◆ In relationships: a difference in sexual interest, or a difference in expectations and experiences.
◆ After orgasm losing interest in the other person, feeling separated or disconnected.
◆ Differences in opinion about watching porn or using

exciting sex toys.

◆ Needing to have increasingly strong stimuli and sensation in order to get excited.

◆ After a while finding that having sex with the partner is no longer exciting.

◆ Guys sometimes, or often, not being able to get an erection.

◆ In a long-term relationship a loss of interest in sex for both partners.

◆ Liking sex but at the same time feeling 'blocked' about having it.

◆ Experiences with sexual assault, rape or sexual abuse.

Other themes that can show up when it comes to sex in general:

◆ Doubts about one's sexual orientation.

◆ Not feeling at ease in one's own body.

◆ Not feeling at ease with the gender assigned at birth.

Does hot sex create connection?

In addition to the list of downsides above, there is also something else worth considering about hot sex. Many people end up having hot sex with someone they do really care about and will automatically assume that this style of sex strengthens their love bond. However, it is questionable as to whether orgasm or goal-oriented hot sex actually does promote bonding and closeness.

By focusing intensely on the genitals, especially in the climax phase of sex, both people are actually engaged in something quite individual, fully involved with themselves. There is not that much space for contact with the partner. It's perhaps revealing, too, that people's eyes are often closed at this time.

Orgasm itself can sometimes bring a few moments of feeling at one with yourself, your surroundings, your partner. However, that sense of unity and connectedness can disappear shortly after the climax. You may even have moments of something you deeply long for, but again, the experience is not something that you can hold on to.

While it is certainly common that two people will feel completely happy during and after hot sex, maybe blissful and interconnected even, it is equally common that people do not feel connected with each other at all.

Not everyone is bothered by this lack of connection, or maybe they don't even notice it. Others are aware of a certain feeling of disappointment or disconnection during or after sex, despite the orgasm. But they don't really understand where the sense of disconnection comes from.

In short

On the one hand, hot sex can be very exciting, fun and give delicious moments of real pleasure and enjoyment. On the other hand, it is questionable whether goal-oriented sex and orgasm-focused sex generally leads to a greater sense of love, belonging and connection – something that most people eventually long for.

In the many sections that follow you can read about another style of sex called cool sex. This is different from hot sex in several ways, but it is definitely still sex in the sense that the genitals are very much involved!

Hormones: what does science say?

Although we should be careful about trying to explain things using scientific research, science can tell us something about the role of our hormones during sex.

As it turns out, it is clear that hot sex, especially orgasm, is known to increase the level of the hormone **dopamine** in our bodies. Among other things, especially at the beginning of a relationship when attraction is strong, dopamine plays an important role. It is a hormone that has a strong 'kick' and can also have an addictive effect.

After a (peak) orgasm the dopamine levels in our bodies drop rapidly and the level of another hormone, called **prolactin**, rises. This hormone decreases sexual desire sharply. Whether this explains the famous 'dip' in sexual desire after orgasm is not entirely clear. It may also be that the muscular contractions of orgasm give a feeling of being satiated.

Nevertheless it is known that people, if they are sensitive to it, can experience negative effects after orgasm. It can show up as a loss of energy, or a sense of irritation or a feeling of being disconnected or separate from the partner. Or sad and lonely. Sometimes these effects can even show up as much as two weeks after an orgasm.

However, there is yet another hormone that is important to know about, **oxytocin**. This hormone gives weaker specifically sexual incentives than dopamine, but does have a strong positive effect on the bond between people. It is also known as the love hormone because oxytocin increases the feeling of connection between people.

While often **dopamine and prolactin** play a major role in hot sex, **oxytocin** is more active in cool sex.

Chapter 3

Introduction To Cool Sex

Origins of cool sex

Cool sex as we describe it in this book is rooted in tantra. Tantra is a way of life that originated at least 1,500 years ago in India, then gradually spread to other Eastern countries. Later, in the Western world it grew to include other methods of personal growth and bodywork. Osho (1931–1990) was a major Indian tantric master who has inspired many people to try another sexual approach. The Western and modern form of tantra is called neo-tantra.

There are many translations of the word tantra, and one is expansion of energy or expansion of awareness. Another translation is web of consciousness. Being aware and conscious of everything you think, feel and do, also known as mindfulness, is an essential part of this teaching.

In neo-tantra, sex is viewed as an aspect of spirituality. Through sex an expansion of energy can be experienced, or a higher level of consciousness accessed.

Tantric sex teaches about the union of the masculine and the feminine principles. This does not mean that it is only about the meeting of a man and a woman. The meeting of opposite energies can happen to any two people making love, and ultimately it is the union of the masculine and feminine aspects – within each individual – that is significant.

Everyone contains both aspects – the masculine and the feminine. If these two qualities/energies come into play, a person becomes internally unified and the life energy can easily flow. In fact, it is almost as if one returns to the natural innocent flow experienced as a baby.

There are many different approaches to tantra. In this book, we rely primarily on the books, experience and insights of Diana and Michael Richardson. By examining the understandings of spiritual master Osho from India, together with those of Australian spiritual master Barry Long, and bringing them into their own personal experience, Diana and Michael developed this vision of cool sex. See the resources section at the end of the book.

A cooler style of sex, in their eyes, is an important evolutionary step in human development. The core teachings are contained in a few simple but effective 'Love Keys'. Tantra as a spiritual tradition is a way of life and addresses much more than just sex and love, however, in this book we will be focusing deeply on these two topics.

Cool sex overview

In cool sex central themes are relaxation, awareness and creating connection. To begin with, cool sex means that during sex you are interested in relaxing your body. This allows subtle energies to expand through you. Relaxation does not mean collapsing or being passive or dead – as will be explained soon. It means you do not focus on building up tension and increasing excitement. Also, you are not working towards any particular goal, like orgasm. Instead your attention is directed inside your body, feeling any subtle or delicate good feelings inside you. And you keep on feeling yourself – moment by moment. It is very much a meditation or mindfulness practice. Bringing awareness and acceptance into every moment.

Connection instead of goal

This kind of sex is known to be connection oriented rather than target or goal oriented. The focus is more on "How do things feel right now?", rather than "How can I make this bigger and better, more intense?" And maybe you discover that because of your own inner connection, a spiritual bridge to your partner is created too.

Generally, all movements in cool sex are done with awareness, so this means the movements naturally become slower and smoother; and then you will realize that this slowness increases your sensitivity and you can actually feel quite a lot more.

It might occur to you in reading this: "Hmmm, relaxation, awareness, not working towards an orgasm, conscious movement? That sounds boring!"

When you first experiment with cool sex it may indeed feel a bit boring! Especially if you are already accustomed to having more active and intense hot sex. But the surprising thing is that you can have a whole range of different experiences with cool sex – even intense, relaxed and prolonged orgasms. In the sections that follow you will find more on this. First, however, we will give you some background information about sex that is known by very few people.

What is relaxation anyway?

Relaxing means unwinding, both in your head and in your body. When we consciously relax and soften tensions held in the body, we are activating a part of the nervous system called the parasympathetic nervous system. This benefits the immune system and increases the sense of well-being.

The revitalizing response is the opposite to what happens when the sympathetic nervous system is activated – our 'fight-or-flight' or stress response. Our busy and hectic modern lifestyles cause the sympathetic nervous system to get overactivated.

So, a simple way to stimulate the beneficial relaxation response, for example, is to do some slow and deep breathing. Relaxation can happen in many ways: by stretching out on the couch watching TV, lounging in bed with some music, after exercising, practicing yoga, hanging out with friends in the pub, walking outside in nature. And deep slow breathing is always a plus, whatever you are involved in.

When we talk about cool relaxation in a sexual context, we

definitely don't mean a kind of lethargy or drowsiness. We are talking about a kind of relaxation where you are really present, your attention is very much 'here' in the moment. It is an alert form of relaxation. You are both alert and relaxed; feeling intensely alive.

Relaxation means softening and widening any tensions you notice. For example, tightness in the shoulders, jaw, belly and feet. And you relax these tense parts again and again, softening the body. In addition to deep breathing, caressing, touch and massage can help promote relaxation.

Additionally, cool sex is itself a great way to relax. Cool sex as we describe it in this book naturally leads to deeper relaxation. Through cool sex you will discover that there is not just one level of relaxation, there are many layers to relaxation, from superficial to very deep.

Two phases in sex

There are two phases in sex that can be distinguished from each other. Most people are only aware of the first stage and believe that this is all that sex can offer. However, much more is possible! We will describe these two phases here. (Fig. 1).

When you are sexually attracted to someone, certain parts (glands) of your brain are stimulated. Your sex hormones come into play and prepare your body to have sex. There is a flow from above (brain) to below (genitals). In most cases, this leads to an increase in excitement and tension that gives the urge for the discharge of orgasm.

In men this increase in excitement is usually followed by ejaculation of fluids that contain sperm cells. In this way a new life can be created – or in other words, the potential to create a child. We therefore call it the biological phase. Most people are accustomed to this type of hot sex with a climax and do not know that, in addition to cuddling and caressing, there is also another option in sex.

It is possible – through relaxation – not to discharge and release your sexual energy. Instead you can choose to keep it in your body and retain vital energy. The sexual/life energy – when not expelled through orgasm – gradually finds its own way upwards, and rises to return to its source in the brain.

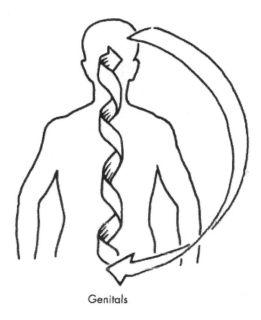

Genitals

Fig. 1 Complete sexual energy circle with redirected sexual energy spiraling through energy centers

This 'recycling' usually results in more life and vitality in the body, more clarity in the mind and more creativity. There is often also the experience of feeling a strong sense of love, connection and bonding. In this way too, we could say that new life is created! More life, energy and vitality within you. It's called the spiritual phase, or the generative phase of sex. In cool sex this second aspect of the sexual energy is explored.

Flow from + plus to - minus

With hot sex, you use excitement and tension to build up your sexual energy. You do this through, for example, wearing erotic clothes, French (tongue) kissing, caressing, stimulation, repetitive movement, using exciting words, and so on. In cool sex the intention is to be as relaxed as possible so that energy spreads, rather than building sensation and tension to a peak, and then losing or expelling it in orgasm.

In cool sex one of the things you can do is to build vitality/energy by using the 'power poles' that are present in each body. Energy usually flows from a plus/positive pole to a minus/negative pole, as in physics: a + to a -. People also, like a magnet, and like planet earth, have plus and minus poles in their (energy) body. (Fig. 2).

Physically (and energetically) a woman's breasts and nipples are a positive/plus pole. Notice that they are external and facing outward. The vagina, including the clitoris, is a minus or receiving pole, notice that the vagina is facing inward. For a guy, his plus or giving pole is the penis, and it's facing outward, while his minus or receiving pole is in his chest and heart area.

The words plus/positive and minus/negative used here have absolutely nothing to do with less or more. They are used to simply indicate the two qualities – one of giving/flowing – the other of receiving/absorbing. If energy is initiated or raised in the positive pole, at some point there will naturally be a response in the negative pole. This is similar to what happens with a magnet.

To bring a girl into a deeper flow of sexual energy, attention should be placed initially (at first) on her positive pole. In other words – the breasts and nipples. These parts can be given gentle loving attention with care, rather than touches that try to stimulate. When the female body is awakened here, and after some time, there is likely to be some kind of vibrational resonance response experienced, as an opening/awakening in the minus pole – especially the vagina.

For a guy, it's the other way around. His penis, especially at the root or base of it – the perineum (the area between the scrotum and anus) – is the positive or giving/flowing pole. If this area is given attention with loving care and non-stimulating touches, energy/vitality awakens and then flows toward the negative pole – his heart area. This will naturally make him more open-hearted, present and in love with his partner.

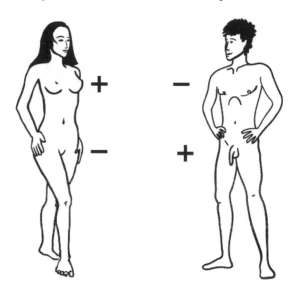

Fig. 2 Male and female bodies showing opposite polarities within

Circle of energy

In fact, when we speak of these power poles, we are not only talking about the bringing together of the male (giving) and female (receiving) that is possible between two people. Very importantly, this magnetic flow is actually something that happens within every human being's body.

A girl naturally gives/radiates from her heart and then this energy or vitality flows toward or resonates in her genitals. A guy naturally gives/radiates from his penis, and then the energy or vitality will flow toward or resonate in his heart area.

If the two of them are aware of this polarity when together, it opens up the possibility that energy can flow in a circle. This cannot be made into a goal though, it is more of an outcome. Also, you cannot expect it, it's more that you put yourselves in the situation, bring the bodies together, and let things unfold in an easygoing way. Whatever happens the experience is likely to be interesting and fulfilling in some way.

For me, it's different

It is possible that you personally feel that in your own body this magnetism works in a different way. Maybe as a guy you feel your heart definitely opens up first, or as a girl your vagina opens up very easily. You don't need to take the plus and minus model too seriously, it is more of an orientation. None of the information given in this book should be taken as strict rules; the key is to be playful and find out what works well for you!

Basic principles apply to everyone

In tantra, sexual intercourse between two different genders (man-woman) is seen as a way to circulate energy, by creating a flow through the meeting of opposite poles. In cases of intimate or sexual interactions with someone of the same gender there is a different situation with the positive and negative poles. Even so there are still many kinds of ways for cool sex to be explored.

Firstly, it is about relaxation and being aware of what you are thinking, doing and feeling, being in connection with one another, conscious touch, deep breathing and being in the here and now. You are present, and not ahead of yourself working towards a goal or specific outcome.

Secondly, it is good to remember that in the end cool sex is ultimately about uniting the male and female energies that exist within the individual. So eventually it comes down to the relationship of each person to themselves, the inner connection to their body, and their own plus/minus poles. This applies for anyone, regardless of their sexual orientation or gender identification.

To experiment with this, you can turn your attention to the energy and aliveness within yourself. Start by focusing on what for you feels as the positive pole in your body, and after a while you may get the feeling of the flow from + to - (plus to minus). In being together with a partner you can find all kinds of creative ways to feel, explore and play with the poles in your bodies.

Asexual

A small proportion of people (about 1%) consider themselves as asexual. Asexual people say they don't have sexual feelings, that they do not want to have sex, or they don't feel the need for it. However, they can still have amorous feelings, have a need for intimacy, body-skin contact and love. Although for some asexual people cool sex would be just as uninteresting to them as hot sex, for others, it might be an acceptable and possibly even enjoyable form of sexual exchange. Especially for couples where one partner is asexual, this form of sex might be a good middle way or path to explore.

Transgender

A 'cisgender' person is one of the terms used to describe someone whose gender identity matches the sex that they were assigned at birth. However, as we mentioned earlier, some people do not identify with the gender of the body in which they are born.

A transgender person is one whose gender identity does not correspond to the sex they were assigned at birth.

For transgender people the polarity aspect can be very interesting. What happens to your + and - pole areas if you change from a woman to a man, or from man to woman?

But whatever your gender was, is, or will be, relaxation, awareness, breathing and all the tips given in this book can definitely open new doors to sexual experience.

Conscious and present – what's this?

As you will notice we regularly use the terms to be conscious or to be present. You might think these are vague concepts, but in fact, they are very empowering. Being 'conscious' means that instead of being mechanical and on auto-pilot – you are a witness to yourself, you are observing yourself. You are aware and mindful, conscious of what is going on inside you, what you feel and where you feel it.

When you are 'present' you are alert to the moment, aware of what you think, feel and do. In other words, you are in touch with, or get what is going on inside you and your body, moment by moment. And this will make you more present to what is happening outside of you.

When you are conscious and present as you do things, you will find that you slow down. You will be more relaxed. You direct your attention to what is happening now – in the present – and avoid getting lost in thought. Most of our thoughts are about something already in the past. Or something hopefully happening, or hopefully not happening, in the future.

Incorporating these two qualities of being more conscious and present, in the here and now, will usually help you to feel more connected with your body. You can sense the body on a deeper level and your experiences are more intense. Intense in a cool way, not in an explosive way!

Exercise: Deep Relaxation

Lie on your back and focus first of all on your breathing.
For a full breath, when you inhale, allow the breath to expand your abdomen first, and then follow with expanding and filling your chest.

On the exhale allow your abdomen to draw in first, and then follow by emptying your chest. Quietly breathe in and out in this way for a while.

Now focus on your body. You can contract and relax your different body parts, one by one. Start by bringing your attention to your feet. Breathe in, and while you do this, tense up your feet. Hold the contraction for a moment.

Then as you exhale, release the contraction. When you exhale, let the exhale/out breath start at your feet – almost as though you are breathing out through your feet.

As you release, you can say to yourself, "I relax my feet, my feet are completely relaxed."

Repeat this process of contraction and release, in conjunction with the breath, quietly breathing into one area at a time – your legs, your buttocks, your pelvis and genitals, your stomach, your chest area, your shoulders, your arms, your hands, your jaw and your face.

Focus on tightening each body part while the rest of your body remains relaxed.

To finish, tighten your entire body several times, contracting and then releasing and then let yourself relax completely.

This is also a good exercise if you are having sleeping difficulties.

What is needed?

The energy of cool sex is subtle, fine and delicate, so not everyone can tune into it right away. To feel this level requires sensitivity and a good degree of awareness in your body. Subtle energy is easier to tune into when you are relaxed, feel good and well in the body. People often hold tension, unconsciously, in the area of the pelvis and the genitals. This contraction or tightness actually impedes and reduces the flow and circulation of sexual or life energy.

Fortunately, it is possible to learn to relax and release tensions, for example through dance, bodywork, massage or yoga. This book also suggests a number of exercises that can help to develop a higher level of sensitivity. In addition, engaging in cool sex itself will help you to feel more present and sensitive, more easily able to tune into the good, lovely and sweet feelings in your body.

In Chapter 6 we will give an overview of how cool sex can be practiced. But before we do that, we will first give more details about the bodies and sexual energy of girls/women (Chapter 4), and then that of boys/men (Chapter 5).

It's possible that you don't consider yourself specifically as a girl or a boy, but that you feel more like gender fluid. In this case you can read the information about both girls and guys and just feel what fits you the best.

Exercise: Scan Body for Tensions

To start feeling more present in your body it can help to regularly do a body-scan. Several times a day, and even right now, simply focus your attention on your body. Breathe slowly and deeply and bring your awareness inside and scan your whole body. Notice what places in your body your attention is drawn to. Do you feel tension somewhere? Breathe into those places, see if you can feel your body without any judgment. And, if you can, relax and soften any tense parts you notice, little by little. If you do conscious scanning and relaxing regularly during your day (and when having sex) soon it will become an instinctive response whenever you 'remember' your body.

Active exercises to increase energy flow

Apart from sex, there are many ways that you can learn to increase the feeling of vitality and aliveness in your body. You can also use other movement practices. It's worth searching for exercises and (active) meditations that you can do at home. Many can be found on the Internet (YouTube).

For example, the Osho Kundalini Meditation done to music is invigorating and relaxing.

Outline of this 60 minute meditation:

For the first 15 minutes stand with your feet firmly on the ground (don't move them), and shake and vibrate your body, including the pelvis.

Then you dance freely for 15 minutes, moving your body in a way that you enjoy.

And then for the next 15 minutes you sit down on a cushion with a straight spine. Or you stand completely still without moving.

And for the last 15 minutes you lie down on your back. Or continue to sit if you prefer.

Afterwards you are likely to feel more awake, fresh and energized.

There is also a series of short exercises commonly known as 'The Five Tibetans'. These are five simple yoga stretch-type exercises (called rites) that take about 7–20 minutes, depending on how many repetitions of each rite you do. If you do them on a daily basis, they increase body awareness, vitality, and your level of relaxation. On the Internet (YouTube) you can find several videos in which these exercises are demonstrated. These are presented in the book *Ancient Secret of the Fountain of Youth* by Peter Kelder. See the resources section at the end of the book.

Practicing mindfulness during your day

Not only in bed, but in many other activities too, our approach can be hot (goal focused) or cool (connection focused). Whatever you do during your day try to be more aware of your body. For example, tune in to your body and posture as you eat, as you walk, as you sit at the computer, as you're texting, and this mindfulness will bring an entirely different quality to the experience. You will find yourself more present, more sensitive, more open, more peaceful.

Dancing with mindfulness

Dancing can easily become a very purposeful activity. Consciously or unconsciously people might be focused on attracting someone, or getting someone to go to bed with them. Nightclubs and dancing are maybe not for everyone, but these occasions can also take place in a context of connection and sincere interest in another person. In this case, your attention is with your body and your movements – sensing what is happening now – in the present moment.

You can reflect on how it is for you when you are actually at a nightclub or at a party. Are you thinking about what you would like to have happen during (or after) going out? Are you more goal oriented or more connection oriented? Are you aware of how your body really feels when dancing, or are you more in your head, more mechanical in your movements? Perhaps your attention is caught up with thoughts about what others might think of you?

If that's the case, you can experiment while you are dancing to completely focus on your bodily experience. Bring your awareness into your feet, your legs, pelvis and heart and feel what that is like. You attempt to be more inside your body, less involved and caught up with your thoughts. What do you notice with this mindful approach to dancing?

Chapter 4

The Secret Of Girls

Every female body is capable of having heightened sexual experiences. Yet not every girl's sex life is only a story of enjoyment and fun. Many girls also know that pain can be associated with sex. This can be physical pain but also emotional pain, for example, due to being forced to have sex. Or perhaps the emotional pain that can result from not feeling much during sex, or not reaching an orgasm.

Some important keys to having subtle and deep sexual experiences for a girl are relaxation, softness and receptivity. That statement might paint a picture quite opposite to the current prevailing image of the ideal lover in bed. Isn't that more the image of an active, moving, groaning sex kitten?

It is debatable whether this sexy approach actually works well for having deeply satisfying loving sex. The power of female sexuality lies precisely in softness (as opposed to hardness/tightened body), receptivity, and relaxation. Definitely receptivity does not mean passivity! It does not mean to be dead and switched off. Receptivity is a powerful force where the body widens energetically and vitality expands and spreads. Out of this relaxed state it can happen that pure wildness arises – a spontaneous innocent natural flowing force emerging from within.

As a girl, if you can relax comfortably with ease and bodily presence, the quality of receptivity will happen naturally. In this way, without any striving, tension or pressure, you will be able to enjoy fulfilling sex more easily.

Attention on your breasts

To practice relaxation and awakening to yourself, as a girl, it is of key importance to pay attention to your breasts and nipples. Remember, the breasts are indeed your positive pole and therefore play a central role in opening the female body – on a deeper level – as explained in Chapter 3.

You can, for example, be with your breasts during the day, having them as your main area of body awareness or focus. Or you can specifically meditate on the breasts, as described below.

Exercise: Tuning into your Breasts

To do this, lie on your back and cradle your breasts gently with your hands. Then lift them upwards a few centimeters, using a slightly circular motion, so you are drawing in the tissues from the sides and beneath the breasts. Be sure that your arms are resting in a relaxed way as you hold your breasts. (If the arms get uncomfortable at any point, then place a pillow under each elbow to raise and support them.)

Then breathe deeply and relax, and bring your attention to the inside of your breasts and nipples, and the heart area. The idea is to inwardly melt and unite with your breasts. To get a feel of them from the inside. So, it's not a focus or concentration outwardly on the breasts, but rather inwardly connecting and feeling yourself.

You can do this for 15–20 minutes or so, every day if you like. For example: just before you go to sleep, or at any time when you are simply relaxing, or as a preparation for lovemaking.

Massage and breast care

In the morning after showering you can massage your breasts with lotion or cream using circular and inward lifting motions. When you give loving attention to your breasts you will naturally open your chest and heart area. In this gentle way, sexual energy in your entire body will flow more easily.

They are perfect!

It may be that you do not feel satisfied with your breasts and are afraid or concerned that they are not beautiful, not big enough, too big, or not firm enough. Even so, we suggest that you do this meditation and breast care anyway, because breasts are an important energy center, and not just physical and external.

Important to realize is that if you are satisfied, accepting and loving of your breasts, then the happier, more alive and responsive your breasts will be. And, if you can accept yourself and your breasts, then a possible partner is more likely to accept you too – exactly as you are. Energetically inside your body the setup is perfect – it's more our ideas about how breasts should look that prevent an internal energy connection with them.

Types of orgasms

Even though we suggest that orgasm should not be the goal of sex, the reality is women can have many different types of orgasms. We mention three types here, but in fact there are more kinds, and they can also occur in all types of combinations too.

Firstly, there is the clitoral orgasm which happens through the stimulation of the clitoris, like a little button at the top and lying outside of the vagina, with nerve branches that go deep into the body. This type of orgasm is often a strong intense sensation, and usually drops off quickly afterward. It is, therefore, referred to as a peak orgasm. Some women orgasm quite easily when they stimulate their clitoris, others have to work hard to do it, especially if they are together with someone, and still others will never have an orgasm this clitoral way.

A second variation is the vaginal orgasm that happens through heightened sensitivity and sense of exquisite melting in the vagina. It also can happen through stimulation of the G-spot, a small area to the front and inside of the vagina. This point can be stimulated with a finger, vibrator or penis. Many women haven't experienced this kind of orgasm. Some women lose fluid when they climax this way, and thus have a kind of ejaculation. This orgasm is usually experienced as more intense and deeper than the clitoral orgasm.

A third type is the valley orgasm (valley instead of peak). This type of orgasm is mostly produced through relaxation and a flow of energy through your whole body, especially the heart area. This orgasm has no peak, and can last a long time. It is described as an intense and total experience, that involves your whole body.

We call it the 'orgasmic state,' in contrast to the usual 'having an orgasm.' Some people can experience this ecstatic state – even without having sex – in nature for example. If you are sensitive to energy it is possible to experience blissfulness in other situations too. There will always be a sense of all embracing one-ness, harmony and peace. These same qualities can also arise during sex.

With cool sex, orgasm can certainly happen along the way, but remember it's not a goal that you work towards, like in hot sex. More about this in Chapter 6.

Clito-what?

In times past, many people did not know about the existence of the clitoris. Nowadays, it is fairly common knowledge that girls and women can often more easily have a clitoral orgasm, than a vaginal one. In our opinion, modern Western sexual education is too focused on the clitoris. From the tantric perspective, upon which cool sex is based, the vagina, especially deep inside near the cervix/entrance to the womb, has lots of orgasmic possibilities, as you will see in Chapter 6.

With goal-oriented, peak orgasm-oriented sex, the orgasmic possibilities of the vagina often do not come into play. Many people think that hard thrusts lead to the greatest amount of pleasure for a girl, but this is definitely not true in every case.

It is in fact calm and conscious touch/contact with the penis, and having a relaxed vagina, that can offer the most pleasurable experiences. The clitoris is a fun toy for an exciting and (often) short orgasm, but the vagina gives opportunities for intense and prolonged orgasms. The situation is much the same with the G-spot. Focusing on it can definitely provide moments of pleasure, but it's great to know the ecstatic pleasure available in the deepest part of the vagina.

Personal experience

"Since a few months I started my new sexual life and I totally avoid the clit. The result is wonderful, my vagina is really more sensitive, plus the area around the nipples, and the nipples also, are now delicious, erogenous, and very sensitive. My new sexual life without orgasm is really a deep satisfaction. I think it's really great to avoid the clit and focus on breast pleasure, it's the best advice I got, my sexual life is really improved and I hope other girls find out these secrets."
(Sharing by girl)

Relaxation is empowering

Relaxation is one of the main keys to having deeper experiences. There are many things you can do to bring more relaxation into your life, such as massage, yoga or dance. When it comes to sex, some theories say it is good to train yourself to tighten the muscles in the vagina, in order to create more feeling and sensation – also for the partner.

However, we recommend you go the way of relaxation. Remember during your day to relax your vaginal/pelvic floor muscles. Do this several times a day. Gradually you will begin to be able to sense and feel more inside the vagina. And maybe the day comes when you discover that sex can be great with a relaxed vagina and bring very deep fulfilling experiences. Another advantage of the vagina being more relaxed and less excited during sex is that a (male) partner will probably last much longer – often too much excitement will cause early ejaculation.

Solo-sex

Sex with yourself can help you to discover what you like, and do not like, sexually, and how to have an orgasm. Even with solo sex you can have a focus/intention that is not only about cumming (orgasm). How is it to touch yourself, without having the goal of a peak orgasm in mind? What happens when you don't build on, but rather relax into, the feeling of excitement?

One possibility is to bring your attention on your breasts first, breathing slowly and deeply and really feeling the sensations it produces, because that is energy, and it will flow! If you do want to have an orgasm, and you know how to achieve that, then of course you can enjoy it. At the same time, see how relaxed you can be in getting to the end. It may be that you do not know how to orgasm, or you may not be interested in (hot) solo sex. See for yourself what feels right, and do not be concerned about whether you are normal or not. Relax when you touch yourself.

If you (regularly) don't have peak orgasms, this might make it easier to relax when having cool sex with a partner, because you are not accustomed to peak-type orgasms. And this can be an advantage!

Do you sometimes use a vibrator in solo-sex? It probably helps you to quickly and easily get excited. Remember, though, that this creates a pretty local (and therefore limited) area of stimulation, and also the vibration can ultimately lead to a decrease in sensitivity of the area.

Fantasy

Sometimes it seems as though hot sex cannot happen without using one's imagination. Maybe you can only manage to cum when you fantasize. That can be good, but it is also worth looking at what actually happens when you fantasize during sex. In reality, when you are in fantasy, you are not in the here and now. You're with your thoughts, elsewhere, and not really connected to your body. Even when it seems as though the fantasy makes your experience more intense and exciting, in fact a deeper and fuller experience is available when your full attention is inside your body, really here and now. This shift from mind to body can require, for most people, the necessary practice and time to develop.

If you fantasize while having sex with someone else, it brings into question whether you are truly in connection with them. Most probably not. The next time you start to fantasize, you can notice, "Hey, I am doing it." You don't necessarily need to change anything, and you don't need to pass any judgment on yourself. This will only make relaxation more difficult. However, you could choose to experiment and see what happens if you keep your eyes open and look at your partner. You'll find yourself less likely to disappear into a fantasy world.

Personal experience

"I actually always used to need to have a fantasy to be able to cum. But I also felt that I was forcing my body and trying too hard to get somewhere. So now I try to let go of striving to climax and relax as much as possible. And when I do have an orgasm it feels very different, much deeper and longer lasting." (Sharing by girl)

Is this normal?

The vagina is a body part that is quite hidden, which means that not every girl knows exactly how vaginas can look. Also, the slang words used for vagina, in English and many other languages, are used as insults.

For children, it is easy to say that boys have a penis, but what girls have is often not as easy to say. The ancient language of tantra, called Sanskrit, has a nice word for the vagina: the yoni. Loosely translated it means sacred place.

Remember that there are as many different types of vagina as there are women. Pornographic images often show a very tight and trimmed vagina, but in reality most are not that organized or neat in appearance. The vaginal lips (labia) in particular, come in many types, lengths and colors, just as the penis can be of many shapes, sizes and colors. As will be explained in Chapter 6, in cool sex the focus is not on a vagina being tight or trim. With a relaxed and open vagina there is more possibility for energy flow!

Sexual hygiene

Assuming a body is healthy, it is best if the vagina is washed with water only (without soap) every day. A healthy lifestyle (healthy eating, not smoking, exercising, having a healthy sexual relationship) contributes to having a healthy vagina. Intimate fragrance sprays are totally unnecessary. If you know you are going to have sex then it's a good idea, if possible, to wash beforehand.

Stored tensions

Sometimes there can be residual pain, or tension, in a girl or woman's vagina caused by having had traumatic or unpleasant sexual experiences. These may have included, for example, unwanted touch, uncomfortable sex, rape or sexual abuse. It is also possible, strangely enough, that a girl can (unconsciously) carry a 'charge' from the negative sexual experiences of her mother or grandmother. It is understood that some patterns can be transferred via the family line, and this can include the pain and tension of unresolved feelings related to sex.

Stored tension and pain can cause a girl or woman to be less sensitive inside the vagina. Many people believe that the vagina is basically more or less insensitive, and this is why it is especially good for a girl to focus on the clitoris for her ultimate pleasure. However, if the vagina is relaxed and free of pain and stress, then this is the area – especially deep inside – where endless pleasure and delight can be experienced.

Chapter 6 contains important information about how vaginal tensions can be released through cool sex.

Oh, no, my period...

Periods are viewed by many people, both women and men, as a nuisance that has a negative impact on the mood and physical condition of a girl or woman. However, the natural beauty of menstruation is the fact that this enables (almost) every woman to create new life, every month.

The time of ovulation (two weeks before menstruation) can be seen as a time of vital strength. Some girls and women, when they ovulate, can actually feel it happening. Others feel particularly attractive and have more interest in sex and togetherness at that time. Menstruation itself can actually be seen as a time of letting go, of cleansing and starting over again, with a clean slate. Having your period (or moon) can be viewed in a positive way.

There is nothing wrong with having sex during a period, it is more a matter of personal choice if you (and your partner) feel comfortable with the situation.

Contraceptives

It's important to use a contraceptive that suits you to avoid STDs (sexually transmitted diseases) and pregnancies. Make sure you are properly informed about the options to protect yourself. Talk to a doctor or gynecologist to find out what is most suitable for you personally, as there are several methods to choose from.

In no way minimize, or underestimate the possibility of pregnancy, if you don't want this yet. It can happen very easily! Although it is possible to have an abortion, this can be a very significant event and one that, for some girls (and guys), can have difficult emotional consequences that last a long time.

Only have sex with someone if you find that you are ready for it. Using contraceptives takes a lot of worry and concern out of the situation, and being protected will often increase your relaxation and openness to sex.

Social norms and pressures

Girls today have to contend with the strong beauty myth and ideal that is put forth, especially in the media. As a girl or woman, sometimes it looks like it's expected that you be skinny, forever young, unwrinkled, with firm breasts, a tight vagina and labia that are neat and narrow. It requires considerable strength to not be swayed and influenced by such standards and to be happy with yourself as you are. Fortunately, there are also counter-movements that are body positive, and confront these so-called beauty myths.

What you can do yourself, for example, is to notice if/when you begin to be rigid or extreme in relation to your diet or appearance. You can also attempt to be more careful of comments you make to other (younger) girls, also take more care with what you share on social media. Problems for an individual can often start with a careless negative comment by someone (or an uncaring sexual experience) – relating to weight or appearance for example. When it comes to sex there are conflicting standards for girls: if you have a lot of sex with different partners – you're 'easy game' or a bit 'loose'– but if you do not want sex – then you're a tease or uptight. Again, the challenge is to not be influenced by outside pressure and to make the choices that are important to you, for yourself.

Insecurities

You could be wondering if your body is attractive enough? Or if your breasts are nice enough? It could be that you have mixed feelings about sex – you feel drawn to it but you also feel vulnerable/insecure/afraid. Not knowing exactly 'how it goes' is normal so some level of uncertainty is understandable.

Sometimes insecurity can be due to challenging or difficult sexual experiences or encounters earlier in your life, possibly where your boundaries were not respected. To find support please get in contact with a qualified counsellor or therapist who is trained in a body-oriented approach.

It could also be that you're unsure whether you're straight or gay, and/or generally feel insecure about entering into sex and intimacy. In fact, boys have just as many questions, doubts and uncertainties as girls have, as mentioned in the next Chapter.

Certainly, a cooler style sex can make you feel more relaxed, secure and self-confident with regard to sex because nothing has to be produced or performed – you can be just yourself.

Female power

With cool sex, it is not necessary that you always be exciting and hot. For girls especially it means, above all, finding a way of being gentle and receptive, in an empowered way. Cool sex gives you the opportunity to develop your receptivity – discovering how to absorb and draw energy inwards. From this basis a greater immersion and letting go into sex and love is possible, as will be explained in Chapter 6.

Exercise: Energizing the Pelvis
(suitable for girls and guys)

You can do this exercise on your own, but you can also do it together with a partner, lying side by side, for example, before you connect and/or make love.

It encourages energy to flow more easily in the pelvic floor, genital area and legs.

Put on some quiet music and lie down on your back with your legs raised, and knees bent, so that your feet are flat on the floor.

Close your eyes and place your hands on your chest area.

Breathe deeply through your mouth, inhale and exhale, keeping your breath flowing, especially in the area of your chest and heart.

*You can make sounds, if you like, when breathing: a **soft ooooooh** sound as you inhale and a **soft aaaaaah** sound as you exhale. It may feel weird when you first try it but experience shows that if you do make sounds it can encourage the energy flow.*

*After a few minutes of breathing deeply, **saying heeeeeee**, slowly let your knees fall outward. You do this really slowly, little by little, as slowly as you can.*

Meanwhile, keep your breathing deep, and preferably keep making sounds with it.

When your knees are all the way down, you bring them back up slowly.

Do this about five times, legs opening and closing. They may feel very heavy!

It may be that your legs start shaking, but that's fine.

Actually, it's a good release of tensions. Remember to keep breathing deeply.

At the end you stretch your legs out straight, and continue to lie still for a while.

Notice and feel the aliveness the exercise created in your body. If you have done this exercise with your partner, you can now both turn on your sides, and move into an embrace.

Chapter 5

The Secret Of Guys

For many guys hot sex is very appealing and exciting. Sex can, at some point, be a primary focus. Why is sex so attractive? Apart from the fact that it is a basic instinctive reproductive drive, the moment of orgasm is also special. For a few seconds you lose control and there is just no more thinking. You are out of your mind and intensely present in your body. In addition, there is a release of tension. These things can feel so good that you want to have the same experience again and again. There's nothing wrong with that. On the other hand, it is true that much more is possible in sex than what you might already know.

Orgasm and ejaculation are not the same

Something that is widely misunderstood is that ejaculation and orgasm are one and the same thing. But guys can actually learn to not ejaculate, while still having orgasms. Why would they do that? Not with the aim of preventing pregnancy because this is definitely not safe enough to count on for that!

Semen is incredibly full of life, filled to the brim with vitality. Think of all those little sperms, around 300 to 500 million(!) in one ejaculation, each of which, in theory, could become a human being. A great deal of energy – spiritual and physical – is required of a man to create sperm.

Maybe you know the feeling after ejaculating, that your energy level, excitement and interest is greatly reduced. It's possible that all you want to do is sleep – suddenly you are not interested anymore – in sex or in your partner. There has been a shift in energy, a kind of loss or depletion of vitality.

In cool sex, men are advised to be frugal and sparing with their ejaculations. Particularly for older men, it is considered better that they conserve their life force, their vitality, by not ejaculating too often. For young men too, though, delaying ejaculation or abstaining from ejaculation (even if only occasionally) has benefits. It can avert the dip or hangover that can easily occur after ejaculation. Energy and vitality are retained and the sexual exchange will go on for much longer.

Types of orgasms

Men, like women, can have different types of orgasms. We will mention three types here. In fact, there are more kinds and they can also occur in all types of combinations. In the first place, there is the well-known local genital orgasm, generated by the stimulation and friction of the penis. This orgasm, also called a peak orgasm, is accompanied by an ejaculation. Typically, there is a specific moment when there is a strong peak in the intensity and excitement, that then overflows and drains away rapidly afterwards. Many (young) men can have such orgasms very quickly, while for others, it takes strong stimulation (for example with a hand) for it to happen.

Secondly, men can have an orgasm from the stimulation of the prostate gland, an organ that lies between the anus, and the base of the penis (inside the body). However, there is an art to knowing how best to touch the prostate so we will not go into detail here. In any case, men who have experienced this type of orgasm have described it as more intense than the local genital orgasm.

A third type of orgasm is called a valley orgasm. In this orgasm, you are totally relaxed and experience a prolonged stream of intense energy flowing through the whole body. It is sometimes referred to as the 'orgasmic state' instead of 'having an orgasm'. (In Chapter 4 for girls this was also explained.) There is no peak, and basically no discharge – or outward going energy – through ejaculation. Some advantages of this type of orgasm are that you can make love and enjoy it for a long time, plus you do not suffer from the dip in energy afterward. In fact, you may even feel refreshed and revitalized.

As already mentioned, this non-ejaculation option in no way guarantees protection from pregnancy, or from STDs (sexually transmitted diseases) either, because some seminal fluid can still be released, without having a full ejaculation. Also, unexpectedly, it can happen sometimes you suddenly have an ejaculation.

In Chapter 6 you will learn that in cool sex, it is certainly okay to have an orgasm, or multiple ones, but they are definitely not seen as a goal to work towards. Important to realize is that sex does not only equal ejaculation – many other experiences are possible along the way too.

Exercise: Delaying Ejaculation

If you want to practice delaying or postponing your ejaculation, or not having one at all, you can try the following:

During sex (by yourself or with someone else) you can try each time – when the excitement is getting more intense – to stop and relax your body fully!

Breathe slowly and imagine that the aliveness and sensations spread all around your body, and rise to your heart, rather than having them flow out through your penis.

You can also experiment with seeing how it feels when you do not build up a lot of excitement, but enjoy a more relaxed approach the whole time.

It is very helpful to relax the buttocks and anus again and again, because these areas tend to tighten and compress the energy, and this brings on the urge for a peak.

These experiments may help you to become aware of how strong the attraction to goal-oriented, peak-oriented sex is, because many guys will discover that these suggestions are not the easiest things to follow! All the same, because of the many years of sex lying ahead they are definitely worth exploring, and it is a great advantage to have other options and choices.

Delaying does not mean controlling!

Very important to note is that delaying the ejaculation is not the same as controlling the ejaculation. If the urge to ejaculate is extremely strong, then it is much better to let it happen, rather than to deliberately trying to repress or block it in some way. There are techniques for this, however, we do not recommend them. If the tension of excitement is built up to an intense level, and then intentionally obstructed, this can lead to pains in the testicles or groin area afterwards. Our view is that in the long term this type of congestion is not beneficial for your health.

From solid to soft?

When masturbating alone, or with a partner, you're probably used to using a firm touch and pressure. A firm touch most likely creates more stimulation and excitement. The downside, though, is that your penis can become less sensitive over time. And then you will be increasingly in need of more and more intense stimulation in order to feel anything.

If you want to experiment with cool sex, then it's smart to investigate what you can feel from more delicate, subtle and soft touches. When you are more accustomed to a gentle touch, you will become more sensitive in general, and be able to feel more with less stimulation.

Personal experience

"The idea that you could masturbate without ejaculating felt really weird to me at first. But on the other hand, I also often felt guilt, regret or shame after ejaculation. I tried a few times to relax when I became excited and not ejaculate, and one time I was suddenly flooded by a deep sense of love, peace and joy. It was really incredible and at the same time almost unbelievable!" (Sharing by guy)

Porn

Things have changed from the days when porn was something guys used once in a while, looking at explicit books or magazines. Today porn is very close to hand on the Internet. Watching porn is especially exciting and stimulating because it almost always shows full-on hot sex.

Yet porn gives a rather one-sided view of sex, and there is usually little, or no, intimacy or love involved. It also gives a rather one-sided picture of how men and women look, and what they like in sex. Porn images can therefore best be viewed as something separate from real life sex with a partner. In Chapter 7 we will talk more about this.

Sex addiction?

For some boys and men – at some point in their lives – sex can become an addiction. This can be solo sex, with or without porn being a part of it, but also sex with another person. Working towards an orgasm and ejaculation actually do make your blood boil and your heart beat faster. It can serve as a sort of exhaust valve, for releasing stress and tension, especially if you have many things in your life that you find stressful, boring or empty.

If you feel that sex is an addiction for you, or is becoming one, see if there are other things in your life that make your heart beat faster: sports, travel, hobbies, work, study, having connection with other people. Also look for more ways you can relax in everyday life so that you will have less tension, and thus less of a sense of a need or urgency to discharge it through orgasm. Avoiding certain stimuli (such as porn) can help you to shift your focus to other things.

Even though cool sex might not exactly fit with your idea of sex, trying it out as an alternative can help to reduce the addiction to hot sex.

The other side of the story

The fact that many guys find sex very attractive does not mean that they never have problems with it. Also, as a guy it is highly possible that you have experienced the less pleasant aspects of sex.

You may have felt uncertain or insecure about what may be expected of you by a partner in bed, and whether you can fulfill those expectations. You might have concerns about the size of your penis, or be worried about getting an erection, and keeping it. Maybe you wonder if your body is attractive enough. Amongst boys there may be some competition about who has done it, with whom, and how often.

Possibly you have had difficult or challenging sexual experiences earlier in your life where your boundaries were not respected. To find support please get in contact with a qualified counsellor or therapist who is trained in a body-oriented approach.

It could also be that you're unsure whether you're straight or gay, and generally feel insecure about sex and intimacy. In short, boys have just as many questions, doubts and uncertainties as girls.

Although cool sex is not a panacea or cure that will fix everything, it can definitely make you more relaxed and secure with regard to sex, because in the cool approach there is nothing that has to happen. There is no program or agenda to follow because the intention is mainly about being present and aware in your own body, letting things flow and move in an easygoing simple way.

Who is responsible here?

Well, it's sometimes said that girls don't make it easy for straight (heterosexual) guys. Short skirts, low sweaters, breasts and buttocks quite visible, aren't they asking for it? What is it a girl in provocative clothing is really asking for? For sex? For love? For attention? And what should you do? Follow your instinctive drive and have sex as soon as you can? It's possible that you feel totally fine with that. It could also be that you would do it, but still have doubts or conflicting feelings about it. Does it really give you a good feeling in the moment or afterward? Being responsible is about 'responding' kindly rather than 'reacting' unskillfully. When we're mindful, when we're aware and accepting of our experience, we will tend to respond with kind thoughts and communication.

The bigger, the better?

Does it matter how big a guy's penis is? When it comes to hot sex, opinions differ. One opinion is that it does not matter how long, or how thick, a penis is. The other says that a longer, and especially a thicker penis, has more effect.

However, in cool sex the size or thickness of the penis makes no difference. In cool sex you'll see that it's all about the energy that flows through the penis, and the simple contact and interaction of the genitals, as will be explained in Chapter 6. Lots of friction type (in and out) movement is not necessary and the size of a penis or the tightness of a vagina is not important.

Also, in cool sex the belief that the harder the penis the better does not apply. An extremely hard penis carries a certain energy; however, some guys find in cool sex that when a penis is a little less rigid and more flexible, it actually is a lot more sensitive.

The penis is able to feel and perceive more, and will provide more pleasure for both the girl and the guy.

You can also experience feelings of sexual energy flowing without physical contact of the genitals, so this means it is possible to make love and have a beautiful energy exchange with your clothes on.

Male power through cool sex

It may be that you think, wait a minute: no more ejaculation, relaxation rather than excitement, soft touches – is cool sex appealing for guys? Indeed, you might think that guys prefer hot sex because they are often more goal-oriented, not just in sex, but in other ways as well. Yet there are many advantages for guys. Cool sex gives you and your partner the opportunity, without pressure, to enjoy having sex for a long time, not just for several minutes, as is often the case.

In a committed relationship, cool sex increases the likelihood that the sex will remain good in the long term. If you have a partner who generally has less desire for sex than you do, then the gap in 'feeling like it' can usually be bridged through having cool sex. It's also possible that any existing difference in the interest levels disappears completely.

With cool sex you are not stuck in the familiar pattern of conquest and rejection that often plays out between men and women.

However, it is important to be aware that if you are used to having hot sex, and you start having cool sex, you may not be able to feel that much in the beginning. This can be a real bummer. But don't lose heart or give up because it can take a while to tune into the fine subtle things going on. Sensitivity can definitely grow.

Even though it is often said that guys are more focused on sex than on love, ultimately guys and girls probably really do want the same thing – satisfying sex that happens in a loving way. For you as a boy, the challenge is to be totally there and present to your partner during sex. And to let go (as much as possible) of a goal-oriented approach. This is the cause of a lot of performance pressure – having to get everything right for sex to be successful. There is no real fun in that either.

Personal experience

"As a boy, I think boys and men should be more open to their feminine, emotional side. Every person has indeed both a male and a female side in them. Sometimes guys are afraid to show their sensitive side, they are ashamed. They are nervous about their feminine side but also long to be at one with it."

Sexual hygiene

Like girls, it's good if guys wash the penis and testicles regularly, on a daily basis, with warm water. No soap is really needed. In the case of an uncircumcised penis it is important to roll back the foreskin and regularly clean around, and underneath the head/rim of the penis. If you know you are going to be having sex, then wash beforehand if possible.

Exercise: Energizing the Pelvis
(suitable for boys and girls)

This exercise was explained in the previous chapter for girls, and it is equally suitable for boys. You will find the instructions on page 42.

It can be done alone or with a partner, lying side by side, for example, before you make love. The idea is to encourage the vitality and flow of energy in the pelvis, genital area and legs – a great support!

Inner connection to perineum

In Chapter 3 it was explained that for the guy his positive pole is situated in the area of his perineum – the area between scrotum and anus. It is very empowering to create an inner connection to the perineum. This area (a little knot of muscle) is like the root of the penis. You can feel this by taking your hands and following the muscular/tissue structure of the penis back into your body. Having awareness of the penis at its very 'root' will increase the sense of the penis as a whole organ – a channel or conduit for energy – rather than having the focus on the head or glans where most of the sensation is experienced in hot style sex.

Exercise: Tuning into Root of Penis

To do this exercise, lie on your back with head, neck and spine in one line, with your legs extended, so the feet are comfortably far apart, and not crossed over at the ankles.

Place a pillow under the knees if you wish.

Then tighten and relax your pelvic floor (these are the same muscles you tighten when you hold in or stop the flow of urine) and buttock muscles several times.

*On the **inhale tighten**, hold for two seconds and on the **exhale relax**.*

*And then do the reverse, on the **inhale relax**, and on the **exhale tighten** for two seconds. And now relax!*

Then place your hands lightly over your groin area, so that your hands are lying to the left and right of the pubic bone. (If you wish to get a greater sense of your perineum you can touch/ massage the area gently for a few moments before you rest your hands.)

Then breathe deeply and relax your body, and take your attention inside yourself to the perineum. You can also use visualization to engage the area, imagining a sun or a star or whatever image

---

supports you. Or visualize warmth, light or a color travelling from your hands to the perineum.

The general idea is to inwardly melt, merge and unite with the perineum, and to help you sense and feel the penis more from the inside.

You can relax in this way for 15–20 minutes or so, every day if you like.

For example: just before you go to sleep, or when you are simply relaxing, or as a preparation for lovemaking.

During the day, no matter what else you are doing, you can tune into this area, and relax the buttocks, the anus and the pelvic floor – all the muscles at the base of the penis.

(The practice of connecting with the perineum can also be done by girls because it generally supports awareness and relaxation in the pelvic area. And equally for girls, during the day relaxing the vagina, pelvic floor, and anus/buttocks is a good thing!)

Chapter 6

Coming Together For Cool Sex

In Chapter 3 we described the starting points of cool sex, and here we explain how cool sex can look in a more concrete way. To start out with, below are two possibilities for meeting and greeting each other – through cool hugging and kissing.

When you are in love, it is wonderful to French kiss (tongue kiss) when you see one another again after having been apart. It can be great to become deeply engrossed and hot desire usually arises quickly.

However, it can also be nice to get together using a different way to meet and greet.

For example, try this melting hug in Fig. 3 – a kind of embrace where your energies connect, and interact, and not only your physical bodies.

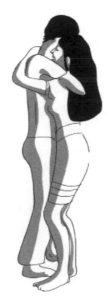

Fig. 3 A melting hug

Exercise: A Melting Hug and Lip Kissing

To get into this, you embrace one another by placing your arms around each other, in a gentle non-squeezing way. Make sure that you are both standing firmly on your own two feet, and that your bodies are completely touching. So, you don't stand with your butt stuck out, but with your pelvises flush against each other.

The body contact should be light and delicate, so be sure you are not pushing into each other, and compressing or squashing your bodies together.

If one person is much taller than the other, the taller one can try to maintain a straight back through sinking somewhat into a bend at his or her knees. Or widen the stance, so that the legs are further apart and the upper body is less tall. The shorter one can also stand on top of something, a step for example, to make them a bit taller.

Then place your attention inside your own bodies, just being and feeling, and not doing anything special. It helps to relax the shoulders and belly whenever you notice them tensing up.

Breathe quietly and deeply together. After a little while you may feel a sense of merging and becoming united with the other, however, be sure that you continue to stand firmly on your own two feet. When you really get into it, this kind of hugging can go on for a long time! And, when it feels like enough, then quietly let go and take a few moments to look at one another.

If you want to kiss while hugging, bringing the lips together in a delicious soft melting contact, without using the tongue, is a very nice connection. The lips should be relaxed and not tense, the mouth softly closed. Then bring your lips together in a juicy sensual contact, and you stay there, present in your lips, and let them melt with each other. After a while you will find that there is a real feeling of being connected in a relaxed alive way. Another advantage is that you can lip kiss for a lot longer, because tongue kissing can get a bit tiring after a while.

Where shall we do it?

There are many places where you can have sex: in bed, on the floor, outside, in the shower, on the sofa. To enjoy cool sex, you need a place where you can relax, and preferably where you have some space. This usually means in a bed or on a soft surface on the ground. If you don't have a double bed available to you, a wide mattress of some sort on the floor can work well.

Warming-up or cooling-down?

When you have hot sex, foreplay is usually considered to be the phase of sex during which the excitement is slowly (or quickly!) built up. The idea is that things need to get more and more hot, that we need to raise the sexual temperature.

With cool sex, the differences between the foreplay and whatever follows later is not as obvious. You remain, in effect, focused the entire time on keeping the temperature cooler by increasing your awareness, relaxation and breathing.

A first step in having cool sex is to tune into and awaken your sexual energy in your positive poles in a relaxed manner.

Female body positive pole

For the girl her positive pole, or energy raising pole, is situated in the area of her breasts and nipples, as explained in Chapter 3 (with a special exercise to tune into the breasts in Chapter 4). This means that in the initial stages of getting together attention is preferably on her breasts, and not directly on her vagina and clitoris. The girl can hold her own breasts for a while, or her partner can also hold the breasts with presence and love, not trying to excite them. Or massage her breasts, lightly caress her nipples a few times or gently suck them for a little while.

It could be that it needs some time for a girl to relax into this, to really enjoy it, but when she opens to the experience, it can be very pleasurable. The touches to the breasts do not have to be strong or stimulating, in fact very often a more gentle, caressing style has greater impact.

For example, see what happens if you only touch/brush her nipples very lightly with your index fingers, or the palm of your hand. Or simply cup the breasts, taking one in each hand, lifting them slightly, and doing nothing to them. Aside from sending warmth, love and light into them. The basic idea is to open the body, rather than excite the body.

Less is usually more!

Male body positive pole

For the guy his positive pole, or energy raising pole, is situated in the area of his perineum – the area between scrotum and anus, as explained in Chapter 3 (with a special exercise to tune into the perineum given in Chapter 5).

What can increase the connection to his positive pole is to hold the penis himself with one hand and touch the perineum with the other.

Or, as his partner, you can place your hand gently around his scrotum (testicles). With your fingertips, which will be facing down on the perineum, use a soft, vibrating movement to caress him there. Or hold still and do nothing, simply feeling and connecting with the area.

If you touch his penis the touch does not necessarily have to be firm and hard. Better is to hold with care and awareness for a few minutes so that a guy feels his penis is being loved rather than being stimulated and excited.

It is true that most guys are used to being touched with a

firm hold and strong movement (taking some care in regard to the glans on the head of the penis) and will say that they like it best. However, a firm stimulating touch can also lead to very fast-paced excitement and possibly even ejaculating too quickly.

So, it is good to attune to a more sensitive and delicate touch because there is a lot of pleasure in this style too.

Condoms and safe sex

If you have sex with a condom, put it on at an early stage. A penis does not necessarily need to be erect to do so! With practice it is possible to put a condom on without an erection. If you are putting a condom on a soft penis, first slide the foreskin all the way back. With a little care, a condom can stay on the penis for a long time, even if it is soft.

Putting the condom on early avoids the stress of getting protection together at a later point, which can break the flow, plus it means that (in case of a hetero couple) the girl can relax and open up without fear of pregnancy.

Keeping cool while warming up

The warm-up for cool sex is actually more of a cool-down. It focuses especially on awakening the body through awareness and relaxation. If in the early stages of sex, you do things that are highly stimulating, for example using vigorous movement or intense kissing, then it's easy for hot sex to be the next step. There's nothing wrong with that, but remember that then the opportunity to experiment with cool sex will most likely be lost. So, the art is to keep an eye on the sexual temperature, and when things get a bit steamy, you relax and breathe!

Sharing love in other ways

Although many people think sexual intercourse is the ultimate goal of sex, sex naturally offers many other ways of being together. For example: kissing, caressing, licking, cuddling, rolling around in a playful way, or massaging.

If you want to experiment with a cooler way, then you will need to disregard the idea that you have to excite each other. Or that you have to climax, or get the other person to a climax. With hot sex you build tension, while with cool sex you focus primarily on awareness, being more present, and relaxation.

So, as already explained, when you touch each other's genitals in cool sex, the quality of touch is likely to be different to the active, stimulating manner used in hot sex.

For example:

◆ You can see what happens when you just leave your hand gently resting on the genitals/pubic area/pubic bone of your partner – this will help them to tune into a possible flow of energy.

◆ Take turns to hold the penis or breasts for several minutes, in a loving non-stimulating way, already mentioned earlier in this chapter.

◆ See what you sense and feel when you put one hand on the positive/plus pole of your partner, and the other on the negative/minus pole.

◆ You can do this to yourself, one hand on each pole, and notice what you feel happening in your own body. Perhaps you can initiate a subtle flow of energy.

It can take some time and practice to withdraw from the hot style, and be able to feel the cooler subtle happenings in the body. When you tune into this fine level of sensitivity, you can have very deep, fulfilling experiences.

General tips for keeping cool

◆ In general, if you would like to experiment with cool sex it's easier to mostly leave French kissing to the side, and stay more with lip kissing, in the way described in the hugging exercise at the beginning of this chapter. The intense use of tongues easily increases excitement and leads to hot sex. Also, it can be tiring!

◆ It can help to have eyes open, to look at each other regularly and use eye contact as a way of connecting. Eyes open also helps to reduce fantasy.

◆ See if you can be conscious of what you are doing, and what you are feeling. And now and then talk about this with each other. Sharing what is happening can be a great support and helps you to be more present, although it is good to avoid drama talk.

◆ You can try breathing in and out together, but you can also do just the opposite and inhale while the other is exhaling. Breathe like this for a while. Experiment with lying close together (even dressed) and breathe deeply.

◆ You can also massage each other and find ways of touching one another that opens the body rather than excites it.

◆ If there is a moment when a strong sense of purpose or excitement arises, you can see what happens if you don't actually 'do' anything. For example, if you are entwined in an embrace and suddenly desire and excitement are flowing through you, experiment with how it feels just doing nothing – and you just relax into it! Breathe deeply, focus on the feeling in your body, be with it, and let yourself be surprised by, and open to, what happens next.

Exercise: Energizing through Breath and Pelvic Motion

As a support you can energize your body using breath and the motion of your pelvis. This exercise can make your experiences during sex more powerful, plus you will feel more alive and energized in daily life.

To do this exercise, sit cross-legged with a straight spine in meditation pose on a firm cushion. Put one hand on your genitals (this may also be on top of your clothes).

Let your other hand move up and down with the rhythm of your breathing, and breathe through your mouth.

Hold your other hand out in front of you, at the level of the pelvis.

When you breathe in, the hand goes up, with the inside (palm) of your hand facing upward, slowly rising from the pelvic area up to your crown/top of your head.

As you exhale, turn your hand, and with the palm facing downward, move your hand back down to the pelvis again. Do this upward/downward sequence for a while.

Then, as you continue with these hand movements, begin moving your pelvic area.

When you breathe in, move your pelvis backward (so you get a hollow, arched back) and contract the muscles of your pelvic floor. These are the same muscles you tighten when you hold in or stop the flow of urine.

With each exhale let the muscle contraction relax again (your back will come back to being straight or slightly curved).

Meanwhile, you continue to move your hand up and down in front of you with the rhythm of your breath. Breathe through your mouth a little more deeply than normal.

*Option: If you want, you can make a slight sound during breathing. With the **inhalation** make **an "oooooh" sound**,*

*with the **exhalation, an "aaaaah"** sound.*
Although you may feel a little silly making the sounds, they can have the effect of giving you a stronger experience of the exercise.
You can do the whole exercise for about 15 minutes. Then relax, lie down, take the attention inside your body and sense what is happening there.

And then what happens next?

For sure you can enjoy being together in a loving way for a long time without actually having intercourse, but this is something that most people at some point wish for. It's not surprising.

In sexual intercourse in case of a hetero couple, there is a bringing together of the male (penis) and female (vagina) which is understood to provide a special opportunity to create unity and love. This, in part, is due to the meeting of the opposite 'energy' poles in the bodies of a man and a woman.

Remember that having intercourse always presents the risk of pregnancy or STDs, and that you need to wish for sex in order to have a fulfilling experience. So, choose what you do consciously.

Knock before you enter...

Below we will speak about intercourse between a guy and a girl. Although most of the suggestions can also be applied in same sex couples – just be creative. When it comes to intercourse, guys often enter a girl too soon. As explained in Chapter 3, for deeper experiences it is especially important that a girl feels genuinely ready to receive a penis into her. So, remember to give time for her body to relax and open up. When this happens, physically and energetically, there will be the space for you to enter, and the sense of being welcome and welcomed.

Preparation can also be done in advance, alone or together.

Through having her focus on the breasts (positive pole) the vagina (negative or receiving pole) gradually responds and opens. When the girl indicates that she is ready, then take time to enter her. That means travel very slowly into her body. The more conscious and gradual the entry is, the more sensitive the penis and vagina will be. You can even make a game of it. For example, you can play with her by postponing entering her, and only when she has asked you a few times, very slowly enter her. This can be a very powerful and delicious experience!

What about pelvic movement?

Once you're having intercourse, in general the tendency is to get more and more excited, to start moving a lot. Sex is then hot and purposeful, with movements that are possibly rather mechanical and repetitive (in and out). This may have the effect of you getting more absorbed in yourself, and using sex primarily as a way to cum, and/or make the other person cum. That may be nice, but remember it's not the only way. It is also good to know that hard thrusts are often not the best way for a girl to reach the heights of pleasure.

In cool sex, you move calmly and smoothly. As a boy, instead of moving in and out (pumping) you can rotate your hips and pelvis in all kinds of ways. This will enable your penis to touch her vagina in a variety of places. Often these more circular round kinds of moves will have a much more pleasurable effect for a girl than just moving mechanically in and out.

You can also see how it feels when you (carefully and consciously) go deep into the vagina and then stop moving and wait with your attention in the head of the penis. This can give you both a very special feeling, as explained in the deep penetration section later in this chapter.

Changing positions is a good idea

With some agility and playfulness, you can regularly change position during intercourse without disconnecting penis and vagina. We call these 'rotating positions' where the idea is to rotate your bodies/limbs around the penis and vagina connection. Of course, the penis may slip out but that is no big deal – you can just put it inside again. As starting out points, you can either lie down next to one another, or one on top of the other, or behind each other. Whatever position you adopt try to stay in contact with one another, via the genitals literally but also energetically – being present and conscious feeling your body, and whenever possible connect via the eyes.

There is a classic tantric position called yab yum or shiva-shakti which is a nice sitting position where you sit in each other's laps. (Fig. 4). This is probably most comfortable if the girl (other couple combinations: the smaller one) is astride the guy sitting on a cushion. Your spines are vertical and this helps to create an easy flow of energy. Additionally, you can caress one another, kiss and have eye contact.

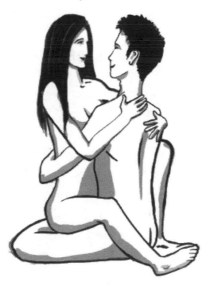

Fig. 4 Yab Yum sitting position

Maybe you've heard of the Kama Sutra, an ancient Indian book on love and sexuality, which describes many possible positions for lovemaking. Although such a book can give you new ideas, it's not so much that you need to figure out in your mind which positions to try out. You're better off intuitively sensing which positions and configurations your bodies want to take on while making love.

To be still is okay

In cool sex you don't move and thrust all the time, preferably. You frequently take some moments to relax and to lie still. You just be and do nothing. Instead you can focus on what you feel and sense in your body.

In the beginning lying still can sometimes feel uncomfortable or awkward, because most people are in fact quite used to lots of movement and action during sex. It is often at times when you don't feel that much, that you will tend to start moving to increase the excitement and sensation level. This might also bring you to the point where you have to choose – to go along with the kick of hot sex, or return to the cool zone.

Yes or no to orgasm?

What to do when excitement takes the upper hand? We suggest: check out what happens when you stop and hold still, well before the climax, and relax! Visualize that your energy flows upward – not outside – but inside your body. Although you don't necessarily have to interrupt an orgasm, you could explore how you feel when you don't climax (regularly). This will happen most easily by avoiding playing too much in the hot zone.

At first, it can feel strange or awkward to not (always) end up having an orgasm if you are used to that, because in that way sex is clearly over! Yet, if you go on exploring, you will discover many different beautiful experiences where there is no real end or finish. Your options will be greatly increased when you no longer limit yourself to the well-known biological phase. You can actually end up having many more powerful and fulfilling experiences with cool sex, than with hot sex.

Returning to the cool zone

What to do if sex gets too hot? When you feel the kick of hot sex building up you can choose to follow it.

Or, if you prefer to try cool sex, here are a few tips on how to return to the cool zone.

◆ Relax and soften any tense or tight body parts.
◆ Massage each other's scalp very firmly with your fingertips. This will bring your attention higher into your body.
◆ Lie down in the spoons position, on your sides, one behind the other. The person who is behind gently rests a hand on the genitals of the one in the front (do not stimulate).
◆ Breathe deeply and slowly.
◆ Tell each other a joke.
◆ Tell each other what is happening ("I'm feeling more excited now") and then relax your body, and be with the inner feelings and sensations.
◆ If you do happen to cum then make eye contact and let it happen with as much relaxation as possible – that means if you notice your body is contracted in any place, then relax, soften and take a breath! Afterwards, continue to stay in contact with your partner and also check-in with what they might want.

Sex with no erection?

Is it possible for a girl and guy to have sex without him having an erection? Yes, it definitely is! You can experiment sometimes when the penis is not so hard. Instead of trying desperately to produce an erection by increasing stimulation, see it as a good opportunity to bring your bodies together in relaxation. You can also experiment with this by trying not to get too excited when you are together.

We call this soft penetration. In the beginning it can seem a bit tricky to learn how to manage it, but with practice you can. For the ultimate cool sex experience, this way is preferred because you literally start from relaxation. And importantly, you don't need to have an erection for sexual energy to flow because energy also flows through a relaxed penis.

Soft penetration and relaxed entry

If you would like to try soft penetration it can be helpful to focus on your own positive pole first so that you connect with your own energy. You can do this while you are lying next to each other, and each put your hands on your own positive pole (breasts for the girl, base of the penis for the guy). Tune in to yourself for about five to ten minutes while you breathe deeply and quietly.

Scissors position

When you both have the feeling that you are ready, it is best to lie in the scissors position or side position. (Fig. 5). You might have to experiment a few times before you get the hang of it. The boy is lying on his side and the girl lies on her back. The legs are intertwined so that the genitals are close together. Your heads in this position will be further apart than the genitals, your upper bodies should be almost 90 degrees to one another. This position may feel a bit strange at first, but it is usually the easiest one to use when you first play with soft penetration. Otherwise you can use the middle position suitable for soft entry (Fig. 6), or find out what position works for you.

Lubrication is needed (and very nice) for soft penetration, so you be sure to have some close to hand.

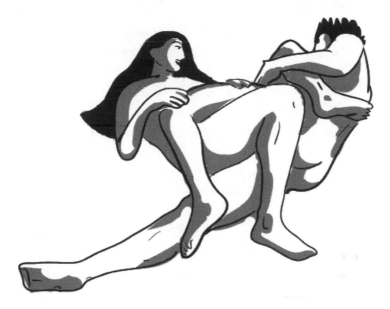

Fig. 5 Side or scissors position suitable for soft entry

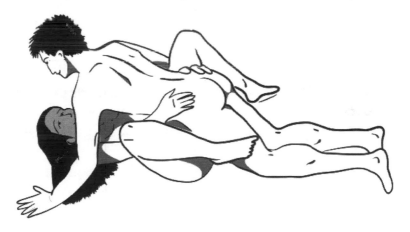

Fig. 6 Middle position suitable for soft entry

How to insert the penis

Usually this is done by the girl but the guy can also do it. Before you start, put some lubricant on the lips and entrance of the vagina. Then slide the foreskin of the penis back (with an uncircumcised penis) or any other folds of skin circling around the head. The girl holds the penis between the index and middle fingers, behind the glans/head of the penis and gently pushes the relaxed penis inside, then pulls the fingers back, and little by little, almost walks the penis into the vagina.

It's very important for the girl to have a relaxed abdomen otherwise the penis will not be able to go in. So, don't try to look at what you are doing while you are doing it! Get your fingers prepared first, then lie back and relax the vagina, and only then begin with inserting the penis.

The first few times are not always immediately successful, you may even need to have a good laugh! If this happens the vagina will probably push the penis out again as the vaginal muscles contract with the laughter spasms. So, give it a go at least several times!

Condoms and oil-based lubricants

Remember, if you always use condoms, use them with soft penetration as well.

Please note – there is an issue using natural vegetable oil lubricants with condoms because these oils will have the effect of destroying rubber from which a condom is made. Synthetic lubricants or water-based lubricants are absolutely necessary.

For protection sake you also need to be sure that the condom stays on during sex.

It can easily happen that the soft penis becomes erect during insertion. This is not a problem, insert the erect penis very slowly into the vagina and enjoy whatever happens.   .

Personal experiences

"The first time we tried soft penetration was really not great. She received the soft penis with great difficulty, and once it was in, I did not feel anything. But we tried it again later and then after a while I felt my penis suddenly grow within her. It was really very special, because I did not feel the familiar excitement of an erection. It was very

different than hot sex, it felt super relaxed and loving."
(Sharing by guy)

"We set a once a week date to have cool sex. We lie down without exciting each other beforehand and then he comes inside me while soft. In the beginning it was very strange and we had a good laugh. But now we are quite used to it all. We usually first, for a while, look at each other and then start to move in a gentle way. We can now even change positions without him having to come out of me. Sometimes we do nothing, are very relaxed and just fall asleep. Sex in this way may not be super spectacular, but it is true that our relationship of late has been better and more relaxed than before. I always have very tender feelings with this way of making love." (Sharing by couple)

Relaxing and being together

After soft penetration, when you are both settled and present to the genital connection, the penis may spontaneously become hard, and then relaxed again, in turns. With the knowledge that sexual exchange is possible even without an erection it certainly takes off the pressure.

If the penis becomes relaxed again, or stays relaxed, first consider seeing what happens if you stay with it, and keep lying for a while, and breathe deeply. You can bring your awareness to your positive poles (girl: breasts/nipples, guy: perineum). You can look at each other and let the eyes meet in a soft way, but it doesn't need to be all the time. It's fine to close the eyes too.

The first few times you do soft entry you may not have much feeling, but if you try it often (and also breathe deeply), you will develop more sensitivity, and this opens the door to experiencing many wonderful things. You then will need much less friction (in and out moves), or even no friction at all, in order to feel something.

Cool Sex

Time to move along

If you started in the scissors position shown in Fig. 5 – a great way to be able to see one another, talk or to be still together – there will probably be a time when you will want to lie closer to each other. Or kiss each other.

Fig.5 can also be with man on left, woman on right - try from both sides. From here it's possible to move to a different position while the (relaxed or erect) penis remains in the vagina using the rotating position style explained a bit earlier.

Many beautiful and unexpected things can happen if you regularly practice soft entry. For example, you may notice that connecting in this way has a positive impact on your relationship. It's also nice because you don't have to get especially excited, so you can join together at any time in a very relaxed easygoing style.

Personal experience

"As a child when I first heard about sex, I thought that the man entered into a woman, and that they then stayed still and quiet. Later I heard all kind of different stories, saw porno and so on so I thought: Oh, you must apparently do a lot of moving, pushing and stuff. Now that I know about cool sex, I think: Okay, that's what I thought as a child, so it wasn't actually so weird." (Sharing by guy)

Deep conscious penetration

Deep penetration is a particular variant of cool sex. In contrast to soft penetration this is possible when there is an erection. The guy gently goes deeper inside with the penis, little by little, until he feels that the deepest part of the vagina is reached. The position where you, the guy, are on your knees and she lies on her back with her legs pulled up high is a good position for this. A cushion or pillow can be placed under the buttocks to raise the level of the pelvis/vagina.

Everything must be done in a very conscious way. If you

enter too fast or too roughly, her vagina will naturally tighten to protect herself from you, and keep you out, rather than receive you inside. This deepest part in the vagina we like to call the 'Garden of Love'.

Pull back penis head a fraction

When you, the guy, feel that the tip of your penis has reached the deepest/highest area of the vagina, then pull back a millimeter. Really, just a tiny little bit. Then bring your own awareness to the head of your penis and perineum, and then remain there, present and without moving.

Important is that you're not pushing into the vaginal tissues, and creating pressure. Instead you are just there – as a light presence. Then breathe deeply and stay with it.

In this way, the plus pole of the man and the minus pole of the woman connect in a very deep way. For both this can be a powerful and touching experience.

Pains experienced in the vagina (or penis)

Earlier in Chapter 4 we explained that stored tensions can be found in the vagina. These can be so deeply embedded that the vagina becomes insensitive or numb. Or there may be points or places that are painful or extremely sensitive.

So, it can happen that in certain moments, instead of pleasure, pain is experienced in the vagina. When a girl feels any type of pain it is essential that she asks her partner to "stop" with the movement. This does not mean to withdraw, and to stop having sex, but it means to stop moving.

It is possible to clear these old pains and tensions so that you can fully enjoy this experience, because every woman can naturally have enjoyable feelings in the vagina. A guy may also feel sharp or cutting pains in the penis, especially on the tip, so he too should stop with his movement when this happens.

Healing through deep penetration

In order to dissolve tensions, very surprisingly, the penis is perfect. When used in the right way – with awareness – the penis has a strong power to heal and cleanse the vagina. The head of the penis, the glans, functions in a way that it can disperse/ displace old tensions and memories, both in the vagina and in the penis itself.

As already mentioned, in a hetero couple, the very moment the girl feels pain or discomfort deep inside the vagina, she must inform the guy and both to hold still. It's important that the guy pulls back one or two millimeters, as described earlier, so that there is no pressure on the pain point.

Of course, at any time you can ask your partner to withdraw completely, however, you can also decide to experiment and see what happens if you both can be with any (often subtle) tensions there. Both of you should breathe deeply, and rest together with the penis staying with the pain point, for as long as it feels right for both of you.

Tensions release in different ways

As the tension comes to the surface, eventually you might shake or shiver or cry. Or maybe you just have to laugh really hard. Whatever form tension release takes, just allow it to happen. You do not need to search for a possible reason for what you are feeling, you don't have to explain yourself.

It will probably feel right to lie quietly for a while, and provided this form of penetration is done in a loving and conscious way, it is in fact healing for the girl as well as the guy.

It might also happen that during this form of exchange, the penis suddenly softens. No big deal. Just stay calm and trust the signal from your body that the penis needs a rest. Later on, it might happen that the penis gradually begins to rise up into the vagina again.

We call this deep penetration because tensions are often

stored higher up in the vagina. However, it is possible that pains can be experienced at any point along the walls, as well as right at the entrance of the vagina.

Deep penetration presumes a great mutual trust and both must be willing. The girl needs to be aware of her boundaries, and the partner is expected to use his penis in a careful and calm manner.

These healing and clearing effects of sex will also happen even if a condom is worn.

Do you regularly have pain?

If you regularly suffer from pain during sex, it is important to pay attention to this. First check if you are taking enough time for foreplay and preparation. Remember that the body of a girl usually opens up more slowly than the body of a guy, so it's good to give her time before entering. Sometimes it's the other way around, that the girl opens up more quickly than the guy.

Also check to see if it makes a difference when you use a lubricant and have gentle slow movements. If you are both willing, you can experiment with the healing possibilities of deep penetration as suggested above.

But if you have any doubts at all – about the source of the pain and discomfort – you should visit your doctor.

Valley orgasms from relaxation

Sometimes there are moments when you fall into a very deep relaxation and become deeply at one or in tune with your body energy. This is a situation where a valley orgasm may arise, you feel as if you are pure energy. You may even sense an expansion of energy that almost feels like you 'extend' beyond your body. These experiences can also feel somehow timeless. This is the orgasmic state, already mentioned in Chapters 4 and 5. This state can happen to you as an individual, or between the two of you as well.

Although there is more to say about the actual experience and the states that arise from deep relaxation, we are not going to elaborate on it in this book. The reason for this is to prevent you from forming expectations, which would turn reaching such a state into a goal.

In reality these experiences arise when you become immersed in the present moment – totally content in the here and now. You can't force it, and you can't make it a goal. Actually, what you are cultivating is the art of experiencing things fresh and new each time, and making love without expectations or wanting specific outcomes.

Personal experience

"We spent some time trying cool sex, but also still had a lot of 'ordinary' sex at first. It was very nice, but at some point, it felt as though hot sex was causing the experiences we were having with cool sex to remain superficial. We often said, let's try to keep it cool. But that did not work so well, until one day we strongly felt that we wanted to do things differently. When we managed to not have goal-oriented sex for a few weeks and we both didn't cum, we felt very intimate with each other. Then, wow, so much happened. Everything I felt was magnified. I became much more sensitive and it became more and more relaxed between us. Naturally there were rare moments, when for example, I still got a lot of exciting sensations but then I could be aware of it, feel the energy flowing in me and yet not get into doing something. At that moment, I felt for the first time how hot sex and cuming could become an addiction and at the same time something that also suppresses your sensitivity. My heart, now especially, feels so incredibly open and beautiful." (Sharing by girl)

How do I feel afterwards?

An important aspect of sex is to pay attention to the time afterwards. Notice how you feel after sex. This will say a lot about how the sex has been for you, especially if you don't feel so good. It's interesting, then, to figure out what happened during sex that possibly contributed to your feeling this way. It can be good to talk to one another, although this does not need to be a long discussion. If you have had sex in the evening, it is also interesting to note how you slept that night, and how you feel the next day. Negative reactions such as a sense of disconnection, sadness, restlessness, or irritation can come up within a few minutes or hours of intercourse. Or even days later.

See if you can simply feel what you feel, and let it be a lesson learned about sex for next time. The main thing to investigate is: if you notice any connection between how you have sex and how you feel about yourself, and about life in general.

Coolness and queer

In this previous section we have written quite extensively about intercourse between a guy and a girl because of the specific penis-vagina connection. But for sure, there are many other ways to interact sexually according to the partner combination. As we have already emphasized several times, the focus with cool sex is not on achieving an orgasm but on relaxation and awareness.

The key is to help the other partner to relax and feel into themselves, rather than trying to turn them on, or to excite them through a more stimulating and repetitive touch. In this way it's more likely that cool sex gets a chance.

Of course, sexual exchange can also happen with simple touches of the hands or using the mouth, tongue and lips. If you want to do this in a cooler way, then let your touches be especially loving, gentle and attentive. Keeping a sense of connection through your eye contact will help you to be more present.

Try to notice the elements that bring you to have an orgasm. If there is a type of sexual activity that you do with your mouth, for example, that always winds up being very exciting and fast, you may choose to do it less. Or for a while not do it at all.

When it comes to anal sex, for many people (gay and heterosexual) this has a strong erotic character and often winds up being too exciting, too stimulating and too fast. That may be nice, but for cool sex it makes things (too) hot very quickly. So cool anal sex requires a strong intention to keep it gentle and slow – and this is definitely possible.

Experiment with basic principles

You can experiment with the basics of cool sex in any type of sexual interaction: relaxing, making gentle conscious movements, being aware, having eye contact and taking deep and slow breaths. An orgasm might happen but it is not a goal to strive for. An important thing with any form of sex is that you do it only if you both really want to. To have preferences about the kind of sex you want to have is your personal right. Be as clear as you can in saying no to things you are not comfortable with, and don't think you should do them just because everyone else seems to be doing it.

Personal experience

"I always thought that normal sex was deliciously relaxed. But now that we have tried cool sex, I feel the difference. I always sleep very deeply afterwards. And then I am really relaxed."
(Sharing by guy)

Extra ways of touching a girl

◆ You can gently finger her vagina and surrounding lips, without strong stimulation, but in a relaxed soft and loving way. Be aware of how it feels to touch her inside. For the one receiving:

feel how it feels to be filled without needing to go somewhere (no goal). You can take turns in giving and receiving. Short nails are essential if you touch inside.

◆ Stroke her whole pelvic area in a caressing way – the inner thighs, pubic bone, inner and outer lips, clitoris, perineum and anus, with variations in intensity, movement and playfulness. See what eye contact brings into the experience during the touching. To avoid infections, it is important not to go back to the vagina once you have touched the anus.

Extra ways of touching a boy

◆ Stroke his whole pelvic area, inner thighs, pubic bone, penis, testicles/balls, perineum with variations in intensity, movement and playfulness. See what eye contact does during the touching.

◆ From time to time just hold the penis, wrapping your whole hand around it lovingly, and then just be with the penis for some minutes, without trying to excite or stimulate.

◆ If, as a gay couple, you want to experiment with anal sex then, when there is erection, start with a slow penetration (with condom and lubricant), and then wait, both relax and feel what you feel. It's okay to lose your erection. Just be very much aware of how it feels (for the active one and for the receiving one) when you totally relax and there is no specific goal. You can take turns in giving and receiving.

When you meet challenges...

Despite the many wonderful experiences that are possible with cool sex, it can sometimes just be tricky. For example, there may be times when you feel absolutely nothing, or you just can't relax, or where you don't feel to have eye contact, or being close just feels too much. Also, the situation may arise where you're feeling all soft and relaxed, and your partner is moving increasingly fast, and wants to cum. It could also be that, because you had beautiful experiences a few times, now you have great expectations! And then nothing special happens the next time you have sex.

All of these experiences are just part of it. The best thing you can do is to be aware that these things happen, that things are as they are, and take them in a light way. You can also share with your partner what is happening, "Well, I can't really relax right now." Stay with what is happening and don't try to force things to change. Very often when you relax into acceptance something new will show up, and the situation changes by itself. Sometimes nothing will happen, but the very next time there could be a totally new experience in store for you.

Inside and outside the bedroom

In general, we talk about cool sex happening in bed, but loving eroticism and intimacy are not confined to the bedroom. Thus, the melting hug described at the beginning of this chapter can be a very nice thing to do regularly. Your body and your skin always desire loving touch, so really, you can never touch, stroke and caress each other enough.

The cool sex attitude of being present and conscious can be used in other non-sexual contexts too. For example: you can make eye contact while talking to someone, or remember to breathe deeply while you are watching TV, or remember to relax your body while you study or sit at the computer, or be aware of how you feel during a difficult conversation, or slow down and chew well while you eat a sandwich, or be attentive as you put your arm around a friend who is having a difficult time.

When you become more accustomed to these more conscious ways of being in everyday life, they will become easy and natural when you are in bed too.

Positive effects of cool sex

If cool sex seems like a worthwhile exploration, then you can put the principles to work in different ways. You can apply them in a big way, and try a totally different way to make love. Or you can try things out in a smaller way, and leave the lovemaking largely as it has been up until now.

Even if you apply just a few suggestions from this book, you will experience positive effects, even within your experience of hot sex. You are likely to feel more present in your whole body, and the heart area will be more available to love.

It may be that with a cooler approach you find more pleasure in sex, that it brings you more inner calm – in and out of bed. In a relationship where the partners experience a big difference in sexual desire, cool sex can bring positive changes that make the difference in interest seem less marked. In the case of people whose bodies warm up more slowly, a cool slow approach, especially at first, is very helpful in bridging any differences.

What if nothing happens?

It might be that, even after several times, you have the feeling that nothing is happening for you during cool sex. It's not special or enjoyable, unless you go into movement and excitement. If this is the case for you and/or your partner, there might be something else needed to help you connect with your body and energy flow.

For example: therapeutic work to heal wounds from the past that you perhaps carry in relation to sexuality; letting go of old patterns and taboos; energetic work; breath work; tai chi chuan; yoga; foot massage; soft massage or firm deep tissue massage.

There are so many ways to support a shift from your mind (and thinking), to your body (and feeling) that can help you to connect with your life energy.

Personal experience

"Now that we have been having cool sex for a while, I feel the difference. Cool sex brings more balance to our relationship. There is more relaxation and peace and therefore also more love between us. Hot sex I have often found great and still do. But if you're having a lot of hot sex, it can also bring a sense of unrest. You can be obsessed with things like: Oh, I feel like having sex and does my partner want it. And once you start up, it can get so heated... Now I'm a lot more at ease with it all. If it happens: delicious, and if it does not happen, or if we stop before I planned, then it's also good. What a relief..."

(Sharing by guy)

Is sex safe if there is no ejaculation?

If the guy is regularly not ejaculating during sex, is it safe not to use a condom?

No, you will still need to use a condom and/or another method of contraception if you wish to be certain to avoid pregnancy and sexually transmitted diseases (STDs).

If it looks like a condom does not really work for you during cool sex, or you find it to be a waste because there is rarely an ejaculation, be very sure to use a different form of contraception, plus take an STD test and agree with each other on how to make love safely. When a hetero woman knows she is protected from pregnancy she engages in sex much more easily.

Ten Cool Sex Love Keys

1. Look at one other often during sex.

2. Breathe deeply and slowly down into your belly and genitals. This helps to be more aware of your body and will deepen your experience. Also, be sure to do plenty of things outside of sex that relax both your mind and body.

3. Repeatedly 'feel' into your own body, look for the small things, discover what you feel and where you feel it.

4. Be aware and conscious of everything that you do during sex. It's about how you do something, not what you do. Remember lip kissing as an alternative to tongue kissing!

5. Regularly tell the other person what you are feeling, your inner body sensations. Sharing simple facts keeps you in (or brings you back to) the present moment, as well as increases contact with the other. Get used to talking about sex and sharing the small details.

6. Touch and caress yourself and your partner with awareness. And use touch that does not carry any intention in it. Discover the many types of touches that exist, from a very light touch to a firm massage. Focus not just on doing it – but also letting the touch just happen and flow spontaneously.

7. Relax again and again. Keep scanning your body and soften any places that are tense or tight.

8. Let your pelvic movements during sex be conscious, smooth and slow rather than hard, mechanical and thrusting.

9. Sometimes start out using soft penetration. If there is an erection enter gradually, millimeter by millimeter.

10. When there is an erection practice deep penetration in the higher regions of the vagina, but only when there is a lot of trust between you.

Possible differences between hot and cool sex:

Hot Sex	Cool Sex & The Love Keys
Builds tension with eventual discharge.	Relaxation and expansion.
Often relies heavily on tantalizing images and fantasies.	Focus is in the body here and now.
Not much eye contact, eyes often closed.	Lots of eye contact, eyes often open.
Friction and stimulation.	Little or no friction or stimulation.
Penis and vagina/clitoris are central.	Perception of total body is central.
Increasingly rapid breathing.	Slow, deep breathing.
Orgasm is the end goal.	Not focused on orgasm as the goal.
Lots of strong fast movement.	Movements slower or hardly at all.
More and more stimulation often needed for same effects over time.	Less stimulation needed for the same effects over time.
In the end leaves you feeling focused on yourself.	In the end can leave you feeling in contact with the other.
Peak orgasm is felt mostly in the genitals.	Valley orgasm in the whole body.
Doing focused.	Being focused.
Ego.	Heart.

It's really important to remember that nothing is black and white, there are many beautiful colors in between. The key is to be as present and mindful in whatever you are engaged in.

(Based on The Love Keys given in Diana Richardson's book: *The Heart of Tantric Sex. A Unique Guide to Love and Sexual Fulfilment*)

Chapter 7

More On Porn

Porn and pornography is briefly mentioned in Chapter 5. Here we repeat some points and enlarge on the subject. Porn can be seen as an extreme way of experiencing the thrill of hot sex. For many people, porn is fairly tempting. This is not surprising as people's bodies respond to sexual images. Even though you might not like the pictures, it is possible that your body might still react with excitement or arousal. Nowadays with the Internet, porn is closer to us than ever before. There are, of course, different types of porn. Name it and you find it.

Pro's and con's

Watching porn can for sure be fun and exciting and can give enjoyable moments. For someone who hasn't got anyone to have sex with, it can be a way to satisfy a need. Porn might also provide all kinds of inspiration for your sex life.

However, regularly watching (extreme hard-core) porn may have consequences and it is good to know these. We will mention a few here:

◆ Basically, the videos that can be found easily and for free on the Internet will often show hot sex, mainly focusing on intensity and working towards a climax of the man. The fact that it is possible to feel a lot of pleasure and arousal with little movement during sex (cool sex) is not shown in hard-core porn. Also, it is good to know that watching lots of (extreme) hard porn might make you a bit numb. You will gradually become less sensitive and then you might need new and more extreme images – every time – in order become sexually aroused.

◆ The bodies of (professional) porn actors are usually not the average. Of course, you know this, but still, if you see lots of certain (unnatural) body types, it may create ideas about how a woman or a man should look like while having sex. Or what they should do while having sex.

◆ Watching porn on your own, in front of a screen, means that contact and connection with a real, live person is missing. For most people eventually doing this does not fulfil their innate longing to bond with another human being.

◆ Excessive solo sex can cause a feeling of emptiness or sadness afterwards.

◆ Watching hard-core porn can be addictive and it's good to understand its effects on the reward system in your brain. Porn gives you lots of dopamine-kicks. And especially with lots of mouse clicks and all the time seeing new images, there is an increasing need to get another kick. For a moment porn can give you the feeling that a need is satisfied. But actually, it never does satisfy deeply in the long run, also because you always need new stimuli. Watching lots of (extreme) hard porn is the same as giving yourself, day by day, a strong shot of drugs.

◆ Porn is simply big business. It's an easy way to make a lot of money, because as we already said in the beginning of this book – sex sells! All you see can be real, but it can also be fake. And in this big business, poverty may force people to do things they would normally not choose to do.

◆ **(Note: please remember that porn with children and teenagers under 18 is forbidden and punishable.)**

Can porn be sacred?

After reading this prior information, porn may seem to be only bad and dangerous. Of course, it's not that black and white. Watching naked bodies and sexual interactions can be quite beautiful. It can inspire you, it can be made into true art, and in bygone days in certain places in the world, sex was something sacred. Just look at the statues in ancient temples in India, or the images in the book of the Kama Sutra.

As explained earlier, it is not about what is done, but mainly about how it is done. Take a specific act in sex, and it can be done both in a fake and non-respectful way and without any connection, as well as in a very honest, loving and conscious manner. So yes, even porn can be sacred, although this probably needs a lot of awareness and growth.

Tips

1. If you feel no attraction to (hard) porn then simply don't watch it. No FOMO needed. Spend your time with real people in real life, and when it comes to sexual desires, use your own fantasies as much as you like.

2. If you feel a strong need to watch porn but you're not happy about this, there are many different types of porn. Select the kind of videos where you're not only getting excited, but which also give you feelings of love and joy. If you want to stop watching, then a period of cold turkey might be the best solution.

3. If you do like to watch, then watch with awareness. Check how you feel while seeing the images. If you feel real pleasure, then enjoy it. If you notice unpleasant feelings (such as loneliness or shame), don't try to get rid of these feelings but just feel them and take a few deep breaths, and relax your body. If the unpleasant feelings dominate, then look for other types of images or other things that distract you.

4. Don't think that you need to try out at home everything that you have watched and seen. In real life, in addition to hot and steamy sex, there is usually and hopefully a lot of kissing, cuddling, caressing, chatting, laughing, resting and occasionally maybe also crying. That is true intimacy. It is good to know that many people have fantasies that can be quite extreme. But many of these extreme situations may want to remain a fantasy, you do not need to try it all at home.

5. If you have a partner and you realize that you prefer watching porn and masturbating instead of having sex with your boyfriend or girlfriend, then become alert. For a while this can be okay, but if it continues over a longer period, it might end up in a breakup of the relationship.

6. In the beginning of a new relationship it might be good, not only discussing safe sex, but also your porn histories. Have you watched a lot of hard porn? Do you still do it? Do you know the difference between porn and real sex? And what are your expectations when it comes to intimacy and sex?

7. Do you have the feeling that you are really addicted because porn significantly disrupts your daily life? Then seek professional help. You can go for advice to your GP/doctor or look on the Internet to find help.

Porn and cool sex – can they go together?

Porn is usually used to stimulate the buildup in desire and excitement, followed by a discharge through orgasm. This can give an immediate kick or high and feel good. If you do it on your own, however, it might also leave you with a feeling of loneliness or shame. If your way of exciting yourself is by using porn, and you later watch porn with a partner to get excited, it could be that at some point this will no longer appeal to your partner. So, it is good to be aware that the use of pornography can have some side effects.

If you regularly look at porn, you can do an experiment

Next time you look at exciting images, do absolutely nothing. Look at the pictures, relax your body, and just feel what you feel in your body. No doubt you will notice that your heart beats faster and that something is set in motion. If you feel excitement and desire you can, just by doing nothing, discover that these can be feelings that you can enjoy – without necessarily having to do anything about them. Pleasure can be incredibly pleasurable when the sensations are allowed to expand through the rest of the body – when nothing has to be done. If something 'has to be' done – as a must or urgency – then desire is often not that enjoyable. When you begin to sense compulsion or addiction in relation to porn, it may even begin to feel unpleasant.

If you are experimenting with cool sex, it may be that your preferences in erotic images change or that you eventually don't even feel a need for such incentives.

Most likely when you are watching a regular movie, at times you suddenly take a step back, and remember: it's a show with sets, actors, cameras, crew, etc. and basically – it's not real. You can do the same with porn movies to help bring things into perspective. Today's porn industry contains a great deal of vulnerable people and exploitation. If you're watching porn it may be worth imagining how the people involved ended up there, their state of mind whilst performing and how they might feel about it afterwards.

Chapter 8

Ten (Un)Truths About Sex

The first chapter started with a list of ten statements about sex that are generally considered to be true – from a hot sex perspective.

Let's look at them again, this time from the viewpoint of cool sex.

1. *To have sexual intercourse, it is necessary for the guy to have an erection.*

Even without an erection, as a guy-girl couple, you can have sexual intercourse using soft penetration. It's a different kind of experience than with an erect penis. It is less stimulating and it can easily be that in the beginning you don't feel that much. It takes practice and tuning in. If you are able to feel on a more sensitive level, then you simply be with the very special experience of a relaxed penis. This can even lead to orgasmic states, both for the guy or the girl.

2. *The clitoris is the main source of pleasure for a girl.*

In order to experience deep pleasure, it is preferable that attention first be focused on the girl's breasts, and not on her clitoris. If the energy is awakened in her chest area, it will naturally begin to flow to and enliven both her vagina and clitoris. Although the clitoris can certainly give pleasure, the vagina has the qualities needed to produce prolonged, intense and deeply moving sexual experiences.

3. *For good sex a guy needs to have an erection for a long time.*

Even without an erection it is possible to have sex (see 1. above). If there is a phase when the penis is not erect, there is no reason to feel uncomfortable and you don't have to stop having sex. Read the section on soft penetration in Chapter 6 for more information. Knowing that you don't *always* have to have an erection can be a great relief.

4. *If sex in a relationship becomes boring after a while, it is good to provide more excitement and stimulation.*

Well, the quest for greater stimulation is tempting. Yet it is questionable whether this really leads to more joy and love in a relationship. It could turn out that you end up needing increasing levels of stimulation, again and again. When you start having cool sex you may feel a bit of frustration in the beginning, because it entails much less stimulation and excitement. And yet it is precisely this way that leads to increased sensitivity and thus to deeper pleasure, joy and love. Through being more connected with each other, you can discover new things in your partner and in yourself – this alone can make the relationship more alive.

5. *A tight vagina and a big penis will produce the most pleasure.*

In hot sex where friction and stimulation play a major role this may be true. With cool sex friction is not necessary. The tightness of the vagina or penis size is no longer relevant. A relaxed and open vagina and a penis of any size can lead to profound experiences.

6. *Foreplay is meant to make you more and more excited.*

With cool sex the goal is not to be more and more excited. In fact in cool sex there is no clear distinction between foreplay and the 'real' thing. If there is foreplay it's actually more of a tuning in and relaxing your own body, cooling down rather than getting warmed up.

7. *If a (sexually mature) guy has an orgasm, it means he ejaculates.*

A boy or man can have an orgasm without ejaculating. However, this requires some experience for most men. One benefit of no ejaculation is that it prevents the unnecessary loss of energy. Another is that you can have more full body orgasms. You also can last longer in sex, and in this way give your partner and yourself more time to enjoy. If sex without ejaculation is something you haven't yet experienced you can start by seeing if you can delay your orgasms. Slow, relaxed movements can help you to stay in the cooler zones of sex where the possibility of ejaculation is much lower.

8. *For good sex there must be a lot of strong movement.*

With cool sex, little and subtle movements are felt deeply and intensely provided you are curious about other forms of sex and take the time to develop your own sensitivity. It is a more energetic level of reality that requires having a good sense of your body. In the end, for fulfilling pleasure and enjoyment you don't need strong movements.

9. *For good sex, you both need to have an orgasm.*

Having an orgasm can be nice, but it also has another side to it. When you are very focused on orgasm, then you are actually working towards a goal, towards something that is not yet happening, so it means you are ahead of yourself. Plus, especially in the final phases you are often focused more on yourself and less connected with your partner. It's good to know that there are different types of orgasms and that the most famous kind, a peak orgasm, is not the most deeply satisfying orgasm. See what happens when you let go of the need to have an orgasm and instead deeply relax and enjoy what you are feeling right in the moment. At first, not ejaculating (as a guy) may leave a kind of unfinished feeling in your body or mind, but the more you experience the benefits of relaxation, the less unusual it will feel.

10. *To have sex, you need to be excited.*

Really, you do not need to be aroused or feel horny to have cool sex. You can make a date to try out soft penetration. Stimulation is not really necessary. In being together with each other like this, a sexual response is likely to arise spontaneously. Or in the case where there may be resistance to the situation, or you can't feel much, you can talk about it and see what happens. If there is a sense of being turned-off you can stop having sex, but sometimes there can also be a shift that gives way to a loving connected feeling.

Chapter 9

Cool Sex: Yes Or No?

Maybe by now you have become enthusiastic about cool sex and would like to give it a try. But what if you are enthusiastic, but your partner is not? Or what do you do if you don't have a partner at the moment? In this chapter you will find some suggestions as how to move ahead.

Difference in cool sex interest?

So, how do you go ahead if your partner is not equally interested in exploring cool sex? Firstly, you will need to accept that for the moment you have different feelings. At some point you may want to share your feelings about this, without blaming the other person.

We suggest that you do the exercises in this book anyway, because most of them can be done alone. Give them a try. Who knows, there may come a time when your partner does develop an interest, especially if they notice a positive change in you.

On the other hand, it could be that you have read this book at the request of your partner but you don't feel it is something you would like to try. Please be understanding of the wishes of your partner, and about his or her disappointment. But also respect and make space for your no. Take your no as a chance to learn more about yourself. Ask yourself, "Why do I not want to try something else?" See if you can share how you feel with your partner. You might decide not to talk about it for a while to give the theme some more thought.

Wrong, or right?

A question that might come up in a discussion between you and your partner is: is cool sex right and is hot sex wrong? According to tantra there is no 'wrong' provided there is awareness. As soon as you become aware, any movement or action will change its entire quality. Therefore, some big movements of hot sex can be tantric as well – if you stay present to each move, and not be too focused on building up intensity (to reach the goal). If you choose to have a peak orgasm, this experience will be heightened by any relaxation and deep breathing you include. It also doesn't make any sense to feel wrong or guilty about the times that you move from cool sex into hot sex again. Enjoy the road you're riding, including all the side roads.

Cool sex outside of a committed relationship?

If you do not have a steady partner at this time, you can certainly experiment with cool sex. Cool sex is not only for people who are in a committed relationship. If you want to try with someone with whom you have no fixed relationship, feel free to do so and see what happens. Maybe the cool ideas don't feel very exciting, but it could also be that you both like the style and say: "Shall we do it again?" At some point, you might even discover that out of an experiment a relationship has been formed.

Personal experience

"When I first read about cool sex, I thought it was really boring. Sex for me was very physical, like, just fuck me. Sometimes it was almost aggressive although I also experienced moments of a more loving type of sex. Now, I'm different from having come across the information about cool sex and my girlfriend and I make love in a less goal-oriented way. In cool sex, having an orgasm was less important for me, I felt for the first time a sense of a deep connection and merging with her, along with feeling the flow of energy and a feeling of great intimacy. Sex can be like a very relaxing game in which orgasm is less important:

Sometimes it happens, sometimes it doesn't. Sometimes we are still for a long time and we just look at one another. While doing nothing there is actually a lot happening. Every touch, kiss or caress, given with love and attention, can sometimes actually lead to an orgasm. Sometimes just looking at one another, kissing or holding hands are all very deep and intimate encounters, which, by comparison, makes the standard fucking no longer interesting." (Sharing by guy)

40 Days of Cool Sex

Quite some years ago, the Dutch TV program *40 Days Without Sex* followed the lives of young people who were accustomed to having a lot of intense and rough sex. Many reported that they experienced sex as fun, but that they also found it difficult to have a committed relationship. Some indicated that they had a kind of sex addiction that involved both watching porn and having many partners.

By experiencing what it was like not to have sex for 40 days, several of the young people indicated that they were more interested in having a real connection, instead of just short-lived sexual excesses or highs.

Yet to not have sex for 40 days, many young people might think takes things a bit far. At the same time refraining from sex is not the only way to gain insights into other possibilities. For instance, what would you think of:

◆ 40 days experimenting with your partner with cool sex?
◆ 40 days focusing on things to do out of bed like relaxation (exercises, massage, etc.)?
◆ 40 days to experiment with sex with yourself using gentle, loving touches that expand your energy and bring pleasure without purposefully striving for an orgasm?

If you really want to try something on these levels, then the best thing is to set a clear intention for what you are doing. If you mess up during the 40 days, that is also perfectly okay. Reflect upon why it was too difficult for you, be accepting of yourself, and then recommit to your intention and begin again.

Stepping into the unknown…

As we said at the beginning – cool sex is a voyage of discovery, a journey, an exploration. You don't know what's going to happen. You don't know where you will end up. You can definitely experience special and surprising things, but there may also be times when the sexual exchange is not very spectacular. If you are exploring remember that for many it will take time, and lots of practice to develop sensitivity before more heightened experiences take place.

Especially if you have lots of experience with hot sex, your body probably will first need to be weaned off the tension and excitement, before you can enjoy the ease and relaxation. However, when your body is still young and relatively fluid, it can be that expanded energy experiences happen quite early on.

Chapter 10

Cool Sex And Relaxed Love

Although sex doesn't only happen within steady relationships, this chapter is about love and relationships, because sooner or later most people wish for a committed love connection. But then they discover that such a relationship is not always easy to find, and to maintain. How do you create relaxed love and also keep sex in a long-term relationship fun and interesting?

The early high days

Usually relationships are the by-product of love. You fall in love, you date and those early days together are usually filled with magic and wonder. Sex is fresh and exciting, and your partner is still new to you, unknown. For this reason, it is possible to feel completely present in the here and now. If you are madly in love, you don't usually think about anything else while you are having sex!

However, after some months or years have passed, the question becomes: "How do we keep our love alive?" Definitely cool sex will bring in a new quality, especially because there is no routine and every time is different, so things naturally stay fresh and interesting.

It could also happen that your relationship started more out of a friendship, not so much out of a strong attraction or love. Then this is a bonus and there is a great chance of things improving, because the starting point was not the highest point.

But the question still remains as to how to keep love fresh in the long run? How do we keep the connection when things get difficult?

Emotional reactions

◆ *He does not call and you go crazy waiting for him...*
◆ *She complains if you go out with your friends...*
◆ *He annoys you because his stuff is strewn all over your room...*
◆ *You're jealous because he/she's talking to another girl/guy and it looks like a very nice conversation...*
◆ *You want sex and your partner doesn't...*
◆ *You want to talk and he does not...*
◆ *And so on, and so on...*

Dealing with emotions

Continuing to have a good time together in a relationship is not always easy. An intimate relationship especially can bring up emotions! Anger, irritation, sadness and anxiety, for example, can sometimes feel as though they are getting in the way.

One of the biggest challenges of a relationship is how to deal with these difficult emotions. How do you deal with that irritation, anger or fear? And how can pain finally become love again, so that you can feel the connection between you?

It can easily happen in a long-term relationship that minor complaints or difficulties pile up – and that at some point you feel like you're working mostly against one another, rather than with one another. Difficult emotions can have a negative impact, almost like a poison, and the question is – how to deal with the poison in a way that does not hurt or damage the relationship?

Suppressed or unexpressed feelings

When you feel irritable, sad, scared or angry, there is a tendency to focus on the partner, and blame them for how you are feeling. You think you feel bad because they behaved in a certain way. Yet this perspective is not really true. What you probably feel are old, unexpressed feelings that originate from the time when you were quite young. This means that the other person's behavior is not necessarily the real cause of how you feel. What they said, or did, is only a trigger that brings old feelings to the surface again. Owning how you feel, and recognizing that something probably comes from your past, is an important step towards having a happy harmonious love life.

I am emotional!

Our feelings can be pushed down and suppressed, and most people are very good at it. However, at certain times everything can get a bit too much, especially in an established relationship. Then suddenly you want to get everything out in the open, get into big discussions, and tell your significant other the whole truth! However, wanting to throw everything away, being toxic and spraying poison doesn't really work very well. Especially when the other person reacts strongly and you end up having endless discussions and arguments that are not at all helpful.

At such times it is necessary to stop, and to become aware of what is going on! To do so, you need to recognize and acknowledge that you are emotional, by saying, "I am emotional!" This is not such an easy step, because when you are caught up in emotion you usually do not see yourself as such – you firmly believe that you are right! And you want things your way!

As soon as you get to the point of understanding and accepting that you are in fact emotional, then you can get to work. Tell the other person that you are emotional, that you are taking a break, and that you will return later.

Letting off steam

Then find a place/room on your own and do some physically vigorous exercise. Go jogging, play football, jump rope, box or whatever. However, please don't put yourself in physical danger (busy traffic) and do not take your unexpressed feelings out on others. Let off the steam by physically exerting yourself. And do this with as much intention as possible, rather than being halfhearted, uninvolved and mechanical.

Keep your focus purely on your body. Each time you notice yourself thinking about the situation that has triggered you, bring your attention back to your body and keep it moving. This might feel like asking a lot of yourself because probably all you want is to get even with your partner!

After a while of moving your body, you can then see if you feel a bit more neutral, and ready to rejoin the other(s). Sometimes it's amazing how even only half an hour later, you can look at your partner with new eyes and the conversation will take a very different direction.

But it could also be that you feel that the time out was not quite long enough, and that you are still emotional (but maybe less so), then this is a sign that you need to go and do a bit more movement.

Totally feeling what you feel

Another option, instead of using physical movement to burn up any negativity, is to sit down quietly and feel deeply what you are feeling. Lean into your unpleasant feelings with a kind and gentle awareness. This is part of mindfulness practice. If you choose to deal with the situation in this way, then you also tell your partner that you need time for yourself, that you're leaving for a while, and that you will return later.

Then sit in another room and focus on yourself and what you experience in your body. It is an art to not run away from the emotion, or to fight it, but instead to really feel into it deeply. Feeling yourself usually doesn't happen right away. Often you need some time to review all your thoughts on the situation. However true they may seem, all of those thoughts (usually negative) will not help you in the long run.

Once you realize this, you can focus all of your attention on experiencing yourself. Become aware of what you feel inside your body – for example, in your belly, stomach, or heart. Try to feel the sensations in your body. Accept that there may be many thoughts about the situation running through your mind, but avoid dwelling on it.

If you succeed in staying with your body sensations, the uncomfortable emotion will gradually lessen and, very interestingly, it can even be transformed into a different kind of positive or good feeling!

You will notice that you feel open and that you can easily connect with your partner again, and the day may take a different turn. The emotion is no longer a disruption, and useful communication with your partner is possible. For example, instead of blaming them, you might then be able to share what your needs are, and what you wish for.

No, you are the emotional one!

Of course, it may not be you, but your partner, who gets emotional! In this case, never say to them, "I think you are emotional." This can be like adding oil to flames. Give them a little antidote instead – a glass of water (to dilute the poison)! For sure it is helpful if your partner has read the section above, and knows how to manage their own emotional reactions.

If not, then the trick for you is to look at what happens inside yourself as a reaction. Do you start to get angry as well? If yes, then you know what you can do, as discussed above. If you don't have any negative reaction, then just be there, present to the other. Take care that you don't get involved in arguments and accusations.

Know that deep down the other really wants love. They are longing for it. If you are able to show them love in some way, or embrace them, that is optimum. However, this is easier said than done because the other person is caught up in emotion, and being in this state may cause them to reject your love. Initially anyway.

If both get emotional?

If you both get emotional, which easily happens, then separate and each do something physical – on your own. You may be able to get together more successfully later on.

Realize that not everything has to be solved with words. Since many emotions are actually unexpressed feelings, they often have little to do with the current situation. However, this is often not easy to recognize as our ego and pride frequently have very different ideas about things.

For a more detailed explanation on the important subject of emotions and feelings you can read: Diana & Michael Richardson, *Tantric Love: Feeling vs Emotion. Golden rules to make love easy.* See book list at end.

Opposites can attract

"Les extremes se touchent" – this French phrase means that opposites attract. In a relationship, there are often some opposites at play. One person is very neat and the other messy. One is very sociable and the other prefers to be alone. One blurts everything out and the other is more of an introvert.

If you're in love, you often fall for that other quality. "He is so wonderfully neat!" and, "She's so nice to other people, it's really great!" However, sometimes after you've been together for a while, the thing that you first fell for gets to be your biggest annoyance. It becomes, "It drives me crazy that he is so neat!" and, "I'm sick and tired of how she always invites people over and wants to party!"

There is a reason that you are with someone whose qualities are different to yours. Your partner has things that can enrich you. For this to happen, you need to recognize the differences between you and acknowledge that you can develop the quality your partner has, but in your own way.

For example, if you enjoy being alone and your beloved likes going out with friends every weekend, then you may have something to learn in the area of connecting with other people. However, it's important that you find your own way, and it might be different to the way of your partner. This means that your way might not involve going out with friends, but finding a different way to develop connections with other people. You might find one on one conversations nourish you more than being in a crowd of people.

Things like this cannot be learned in one day, for some people it takes years before they can do something along these lines. In the case of recurring irritation and controversies, it may be interesting to take a look at qualities your partner has which seem different or opposite to yours, and consider the areas where you might learn something from one another.

What about having sex when emotional?

What do you do when anger, irritation or annoyance prevail in your relationship? Do you (still) have sex or not? Hot sex can give a certain sense of relief, but it can also make the sense of separation between you feel even more pronounced. Cool sex can often feel like a big step too. It can feel more of a challenge to actually feel what you feel, and share it, rather than to just close your eyes and have fast hot sex with each other. But cool sex can provide a good opportunity to start to recover a sense of love and connection to your partner, and to yourself!

Desire, or no desire?

In a relationship, a difference in the level of sexual desire can be a tricky thing. If this is something that frequently causes conflict for you, take the opportunity to look into it a bit more deeply. If you don't really address the issue then feelings of rejection, disappointment, guilt and pain can build up and cause tension and worry.

If you are the one who usually wants to have sex more often, then investigate your desire a bit. Are you using sex to find an outlet for tension and stress? Are you wanting to have sex often to enjoy the physical experience? Are you looking for intimacy, a hug, a touch? Are you so crazy about the other person that you have a sense of wanting to merge with them? And how is the rest of your relationship? Is sex something that is confined to bed for you, or do you touch your partner outside of the bedroom too? Investigate whether you can feel desire without having to do something about it immediately.

Also imagine you are the other person. Do you have a sense of what things are like for your partner? Do you know why your partner has more or less desire for sex than you do? And do you know what his or her experience of sex is, in general? Do you know what he or she really longs for?

If you are the one who has less desire for sex in the relationship, then look at your disinterest. What don't you like? What's in the way that keeps you from having a sexual connection with your partner? What would you like? What would you need?

Also see if you can feel what you are experiencing in your body. Behind your resistance to sex, might there be some anger or sadness about something that has happened to you? Or about what your experience has been in having sex (sometimes)? Do you have a sense of what things are like for your partner? Do you know what his or her needs or desires are? Remember that a healthy body usually longs for touch and physical intimacy.

However, emotions and negative thoughts can easily block sexual openness and a person may not want to have goal-oriented hot sex – in fact their longing is for connection. If you don't feel like hot sex on a regular basis and you try cool sex instead, then you might discover there is much less resistance to engaging in sex. Cool sex will usually bring more balance and a quality of connection to the relationship.

Personal experience

"Previously, we really had difficulties about whether or not to have sex. She just wanted it much less often than I do. But now, with cool sex, this is not as much the case. She's willing to try soft penetration and from that beginning there are always interesting and sometimes surprising things that happen. I myself am now less focused on hot sex, so yes, this affects things too. It really is a lot quieter and things are much more loving between us."

(Sharing by guy)

Exercise: King/Queen and Servant Game

In a relationship you can (unconsciously) be longing for the other to identify and fulfill your desires, wishes that you hardly even recognize yourself. This can lead to disappointment. After all, if you yourself don't really know what your desires are you cannot expect the other person to. On the other hand, you may be concerned that the other person won't like or approve of certain desires you have, so you don't risk revealing them. In this way you might miss a great opportunity.

The King/Queen and Servant Game is a fun way for two people to learn about their desires. To play, you choose one of you to be the king or queen for a certain amount of time (for example, two hours). He or she gets the chance to tell the other (the servant) all of his or her needs and desires. The servant tries to meet or fulfill them.

These desires as much as possible need to be fair. A real king or queen would not want a servant to do something beyond his or her limits. A servant cannot say no to things, but within his or her limits, can try to find something that fits in with the intention of finding a way to fulfill that need or wish. But in a way that is within their own comfort zone.

After the agreed time you turn the tables and the other

---

person gets equal time to be king or queen. This exercise is an opportunity to get very creative with intimacy and sexuality. Let yourself be creative about your requests. You may want to be given a long bath or have your hair washed or blown dry or be gently massaged with massage oil or lotion. Or try using this exercise to invite or seduce your partner into a cooler type of sexual experience with you, even if it is not his or her usual preference.

No sexual interest?

Especially when you've been together for quite some time, and there are so many other things that you need to get done, it may be that you end up not having sex very often. If you both have little or no desire, it's usually no real reason for concern. For some couples, intimacy is to be found in things like hugging, caressing, massaging, instead of sex. With other couples that intimacy level, too, threatens to disappear. If this is the case for you, then cool sex with soft penetration, as described in Chapter 6, could be a good option to help you stay in connection (including sexually), and nourish the bond and love you share.

Stay or leave?

In almost every relationship there will be times when there are doubts. Should we stay together or not? Some couples separate, others stay together. There are really no set guidelines that can address these doubts because each situation, each relationship, is unique.

If you're going through a difficult time, the question is how to manage it? Are you always fighting and arguing? Do you break up? And then make up? Is all the blame placed on your partner? Is addiction being used as a way to escape your difficulties?

What can give you the fastest insight, if you are having a hard time, is to fully accept the situation for what it is. This could be – boring, heavy, dark, hard, hopeless. Try shifting your focus from your thoughts to the actual feelings in your body that go with them. It is helpful to take space from each other to do this, so that each person finds their own way.

What could emerge from this time apart is that you reconnect, with a sense of really wanting to be with your partner – that there is still enough love between you to face the dark period in your relationship. It may even be that after a phase of difficulties, you feel a renewed, and even greater sense, of how much you love your partner.

But it is also possible that the time comes when one or both of you are sure that you want to end the relationship. It often takes courage to make such a decision, and needs strength to follow through. In such a case, it is wise to not see one another for a while, however difficult, as this will help you to let go of each other and give you space to grieve.

It's good to take time to understand what your part in the breakup has been, and important that you know in some way how to address these issues, to avoid the same things coming up again when you get involved with someone else.

I love...

A relationship filled with a relaxed vibration of love and awareness is something that most people learn through trial and error. Give yourself time and space to experiment, with respect for yourself and others. Let your intention for your relationship be a place for love, a love in which both of you can grow and expand.

Last but not least, the first step in loving someone else, is to love yourself first.

Yesterday is History,
Tomorrow is a Mystery,
But today is a Gift,
That is why it is called the Present.
(*Kung Fu Panda*)

Cool Sex is published in the following languages:

Dutch edition in full color:
Coole seks, relaxte liefde. Hét handboek voor liefdevolle seks
Aramith/Gottmer, Haarlem, Netherlands. 2010
ISBN 9789068342338

German edition in full color:
Cooler sex. Das Handbuch für ein richtig gutes Liebesleben
Innenwelt Verlag, Cologne, Germany. 2015
ISBN 978-3-942502-44-3

French edition in full color:
Cool sex. Sexualité plus cool... vie amoureuse plus simple?
Almasta, Switzerland. 2018
ISBN 978 2-940095-42-1

Spanish edition in 3 colors:
Sexo Cool. Manual de sexualidad amorosa para jóvenes
Ediciones Urano, Spain. 2019
ISBN 978-84-16344-36-9

English edition in black and white:
Cool Sex.
An essential young adult guide to loving, mindful sex.
O-Books, UK. 2020
ISBN 978-1-78904-351-8

About the Authors

Wendy Doeleman (1970) has a Social Science Degree (University of Utrecht) and worked for many years as a trainer and author in the field of welfare and childcare. Her interest in tantra began in 2005 and since then she has explored a variety of approaches, including participating in the "Making Love Retreat" with Diana and Michael Richardson. This ground-breaking retreat inspired Wendy to collaborate with Diana and write the book *Coole seks, relaxte liefde* for young adults, published in Dutch in 2010. She offers tantra workshops in the Netherlands, mainly for young people and is committed to sex education from a holistic and conscious point of view. Wendy is mother of three sons and lives in the Netherlands with her partner Remi.

www.blissyourbody.nl

Diana Richardson is considered to be one of today's leading authorities on human sexuality. She is the best-selling author of eight books on how in practical ways a person can experience a more fulfilling sex and love life. Born in South Africa in 1954, she first qualified as a lawyer (B.A.LLB) (University of Natal, Durban), and then she trained as a holistic massage therapist (ITEC) in the UK. Her interest in the body and healing prompted an intense personal exploration into the union of sex and meditation – the essence of neo-tantra – based on the teachings of Osho and Barry Long. Since 1993, together with her partner, Michael, she has been sharing her insights and experiences with couples who travel from many different parts of the world to participate in their informative and life-changing Making Love Retreats in Switzerland, where Diana and Michael are based.

Diana and Michael Richardson:
www.livinglove.com

Recommended Books and Resources

Osho: The Book of Secrets. 112 Meditations to Discover the Mystery Within
St. Martin's Griffin, US. 2010
ISBN-10: 9780312650605
There are many clips on YouTube of Osho speaking on a wide variety of subjects.

Barry Long: Making Love: Sexual Love the Divine Way
Barry Long Books. 2014. www.barrylong.org
ASIN: B00LETUU92 (also available in audio)

Peter Kelder: Ancient Secret of the Fountain of Youth
Virgin Publishing, UK. 2011
ISBN-10: 0753540053

Eckhart Tolle: The Power of Now
New World Library, USA. 2001
ISBN-10: 9780340733509 (also available in audio)

Marshall B. Rosenberg: Nonviolent Communication: A Language of Life
PuddleDancer Press, USA. 2003
ISBN-10: 9781892005038 (also available in audio)

Lance Dane: The Complete Illustrated Kama Sutra
Inner Traditions, USA. 2003
ISBN-10: 0892811382

Darren Cockburn: Being Present: Cultivate a Peaceful Mind through Spiritual Practice
Inner Traditions, USA. 2018
ISBN-13: 978-1844097463
Mindfulness trainings: https://mindfulnessonlinetraining.org

Puberty, Menstruation and Contraception:
Red School: https://redschool.net
Jane Bennett and Alexandra Pope: The Pill: Are you sure it's for you?
Orion, UK. 2009
ASIN: B013JDOUCI

Therapy with body-oriented approach suggestion:
See Practitioner Directory for the somatic experiencing (SE) work of Peter Levine: https://traumahealing.org

Previous Titles in English
by Diana & Michael Richardson

The Heart of Tantric Sex.
A Unique Guide to Love and Sexual Fulfilment
Diana Richardson, O-Books, UK. 2003
ISBN 978-1-90381-637-8

Tantric Orgasm for Women
Diana Richardson, Destiny Books, USA. 2004
ISBN 978-0-89281-133-5

Tantric Love: Feeling vs Emotion. Golden rules to make love easy
Diana & Michael Richardson, O-Books, UK. 2004
ISBN 978-1-84694-283-9

Tantric Sex for Men: Making Love a Meditation
Diana & Michael Richardson, Destiny Books, USA. 2010
ISBN 978-1-59477-311-2

Slow Sex. The Path to Fulfilling and Sustainable Sexuality
Diana Richardson, Destiny Books, USA. 2011
ISBN 978-1-59477-367-9

Tantric Love Letters: On Sex and Affairs of the Heart
Diana Richardson, O-Books, UK. 2011
ISBN 978-1-78099-154-2

Tantric Sex and Menopause. Practices for Spiritual and Sexual Renewal
Diana Richardson & Janet McGeever, Destiny Books, USA. 2018
ISBN 978-1-62055-683-2

TEDx Talk by Diana Richardson – **The Power of Mindful Sex.**
17 minutes. YouTube. English language.

BOOKS

SPIRITUALITY

O is a symbol of the world, of oneness and unity; this eye represents knowledge and insight. We publish titles on general spirituality and living a spiritual life. We aim to inform and help you on your own journey in this life.

If you have enjoyed this book, why not tell other readers by posting a review on your preferred book site?

Recent bestsellers from O-Books are:

The Heart of Tantric Sex
Diana Richardson
Revealing Eastern secrets of deep love and intimacy to Western couples.
Paperback: 978-1-90381-637-0 ebook: 978-1-84694-637-0

Crystal Prescriptions
The A-Z guide to over 1,200 symptoms and their healing crystals
Judy Hall
The first in the popular series of eight books, this handy little guide is packed as tight as a pill-bottle with crystal remedies for ailments.
Paperback: 978-1-90504-740-6 ebook: 978-1-84694-629-5

Take Me To Truth
Undoing the Ego
Nouk Sanchez, Tomas Vieira
The best-selling step-by-step book on shedding the Ego, using the teachings of *A Course In Miracles*.
Paperback: 978-1-84694-050-7 ebook: 978-1-84694-654-7

The 7 Myths about Love...Actually!
The Journey from your HEAD to the HEART of your SOUL
Mike George
Smashes all the myths about LOVE.
Paperback: 978-1-84694-288-4 ebook: 978-1-84694-682-0

The Holy Spirit's Interpretation of the New Testament
A Course in Understanding and Acceptance
Regina Dawn Akers
Following on from the strength of *A Course In Miracles*, NTI teaches us how to experience the love and oneness of God.
Paperback: 978-1-84694-085-9 ebook: 978-1-78099-083-5

Dying to Be Free
From Enforced Secrecy to Near Death to True Transformation
Hannah Robinson
After an unexpected accident and near-death experience, Hannah Robinson found herself radically transforming her life, while a remarkable new insight altered her relationship with her father, a practising Catholic priest.
Paperback: 978-1-78535-254-6 ebook: 978-1-78535-255-3

The Ecology of the Soul
A Manual of Peace, Power and Personal Growth for Real People in the Real World
Aidan Walker
Balance your own inner Ecology of the Soul to regain your natural state of peace, power and wellbeing.
Paperback: 978-1-78279-850-7 ebook: 978-1-78279-849-1

On the Other Side of Love
A woman's unconventional journey towards wisdom
Muriel Maufroy
When life has lost all meaning, what do you do?
Paperback: 978-1-78535-281-2 ebook: 978-1-78535-282-9

Practicing A Course In Miracles
A translation of the Workbook in plain language, with mentor's notes
Elizabeth A. Cronkhite
The practical second and third volumes of The Plain-Language *A Course In Miracles*.
Paperback: 978-1-84694-403-1 ebook: 978-1-78099-072-9

Readers of ebooks can buy or view any of these bestsellers by clicking on the live link in the title. Most titles are published in paperback and as an ebook. Paperbacks are available in traditional bookshops. Both print and ebook formats are available online.

Find more titles and sign up to our readers' newsletter at
http://www.johnhuntpublishing.com/mind-body-spirit

Follow us on Facebook at https://www.facebook.com/OBooks/
and Twitter at https://twitter.com/obooks